YOUR EYES

**Questions
you
have
. . . Answers
you
need**

Other Books in This Series
From the People's Medical Society

Alzheimer's & Dementia: Questions You Have . . . Answers You Need

Arthritis: Questions You Have . . . Answers You Need

Asthma: Questions You Have . . . Answers You Need

Back Pain: Questions You Have . . . Answers You Need

Blood Pressure: Questions You Have . . . Answers You Need

Cholesterol & Triglycerides: Questions You Have . . . Answers You Need

Depression: Questions You Have . . . Answers You Need

Diabetes: Questions You Have . . . Answers You Need

Hearing Loss: Questions You Have . . . Answers You Need

Prostate: Questions You Have . . . Answers You Need

Stroke: Questions You Have . . . Answers You Need

Vitamins and Minerals: Questions You Have . . . Answers You Need

Your Heart: Questions You Have . . . Answers You Need

YOUR EYES

Questions
you
have
...Answers
you
need

By Sandra Salmans

≡People's Medical Society®

Allentown, Pennsylvania

The People's Medical Society is a nonprofit consumer health organization dedicated to the principles of better, more responsive and less expensive medical care. Organized in 1983, the People's Medical Society puts previously unavailable medical information into the hands of consumers so that they can make informed decisions about their own health care.

Membership in the People's Medical Society is $20 a year and includes a subscription to the *People's Medical Society Newsletter.* For information, write to the People's Medical Society, 462 Walnut Street, Allentown, PA 18102, or call 610-770-1670.

This and other People's Medical Society publications are available for quantity purchase at discount. Contact the People's Medical Society for details.

Many of the designations used by manufacturers and sellers to distinguish their products are claimed as trademarks. Where those designations appear in this book and the People's Medical Society was aware of a trademark claim, the designations have been printed in initial capital letters (e.g., Botox).

Library of Congress Cataloging-in-Publication Data
Salmans, Sandra.
      Your eyes : questions you have—answers you need /
by Sandra Salmans.
            p. cm.
      Includes bibliographical references and index.
      ISBN 1-882606-59-0
      1. Eye—Diseases—Miscellanea.   2. Ophthalmology—
Miscellanea.   I. Title.
RE51.S18   1996
617.7—dc20   96-1464
                                                              CIP

  2 3 4 5 6 7 8 9 0
First printing, April 1996

CONTENTS

Introduction 7

Chapter 1 Focusing on the Eye 11
        Eye Examination 17
        Eye Care Professionals 21

Chapter 2 General Eye Disorders and Diseases 25
        Refractive Errors 25
        Corrective Methods 29
        Crossed Eyes 35
        Treatment for Strabismus 38
        Amblyopia ("Lazy Eye") 43
        Floaters and Flashes 45
        Infections and Inflammations 47
        Structural Eyelid Problems 55
        Excessive Tears and Dry Eyes 58
        Other Eye Disorders 62

Chapter 3 Retinal Disorders 67
        Macular Degeneration 68
        Diabetic Retinopathy 76
        Torn and Detached Retinas 84

Retinitis Pigmentosa 90
CMV Retinitis 96
Tumors 98
Other Retinal Problems 100

Chapter 4 Cataracts 103
Cataract Surgery 110
Criteria for Surgery 111
Surgical Approaches 117

Chapter 5 Glaucoma 127
Examination 133
Treatment 135

Chapter 6 Other Questions About the Eye 145
Other Vision-Threatening Conditions 146
Low Vision Devices 150

Informational and Mutual-Aid Groups 153

Eye Treatment Centers 155

Glossary 159

Suggested Reading 171

Appendix: Types of Eye Devices 173

Index 179

INTRODUCTION

Most of us take our eyes for granted. We think little about how they work, what can go wrong with them and what they really mean to our overall lives. If you asked a group of average people what they worry about most in terms of their health, losing their sight would be either low or not even mentioned on the list. That, of course, is until something goes wrong!

As the philosopher said, "Our eyes are our window to the world." And when our vision is threatened, so is our quality of life. Of all our senses, sight is the most far reaching and revealing. Without sight, our world shrinks. It's hard to think of a world without colors and faces. It's hard to conceive of having to use our imaginations and other senses to "picture" the world around us. Yet without sight, that is what we would need to do.

And that is precisely why we have written *Your Eyes: Questions You Have ... Answers You Need.* It is the guidebook to your eyes. It is designed to help you understand how your eyes work, what problems might occur and how to prevent or treat those problems. Our goal is to educate and empower you. The more you know about your eyes, the better you will be able to make decisions that affect them.

Eye care and treatment have been changing radically in recent years. Not many years ago a cataract operation meant weeks in bed with no head movement allowed. Today the procedure is often performed in a nonhospital setting with a speedy recovery. These days there are surgical techniques to treat vision problems that a decade ago were untreatable. We know more about glaucoma than ever before and have developed new and better ways to diagnose and treat it. All in all, the world of vision has grown brighter as new research and technologies have come along.

Author Sandra Salmans has done an extraordinary job of poring through the medical literature and speaking with leading authorities in the field of eye care. She has taken material that is often difficult to understand and made it readable and understandable. I know that you will find *Your Eyes: Questions You Have ... Answers You Need* one of the most helpful books you will ever read on a health-care subject.

Charles B. Inlander
President
People's Medical Society

YOUR EYES

**Questions
you
have
...Answers
you
need**

Terms printed in boldface can be found in the glossary, beginning on page 159. Only the first mention of the word in the text will be boldfaced.

We have tried to use male and female pronouns in an egalitarian manner throughout the book. Any imbalance in usage has been in the interest of readability.

1 FOCUSING ON THE EYE

Q: I know what the eye looks like, obviously. But what is it, exactly?

A: What you see is only a fraction of the eye—there's a lot more than meets the eye! The eye is an almost spherical object, a bit less than an inch in diameter. It's an organ—technically, a dual organ, because each of us has a pair of eyes—with its own muscular, circulatory and nervous systems.

It rests in a bony socket called the **orbit**, which encloses it completely except for the frontal opening (that's the part you see through) and several rear openings for blood vessels and nerves.

Q: What is the eye itself composed of?

A: The outermost layer is a delicate protective membrane called the **conjunctiva**, which covers the **sclera**, or white of the eye. The conjunctiva also lines the inside of the lids.

The sclera wraps almost completely around the eye. It's interrupted only by a transparent, dome-shaped membrane, the **cornea**, that covers the front of the eye, and by the **optic nerve** at the back of the eyeball.

Directly behind the cornea is the **iris**, the pigmented structure that gives the eye its color, and at the center of the iris is the **pupil**. The **lens**, which is about the size of a pea, sits just behind the iris. There are three parts to the lens: the **capsule**, a thin membrane that completely surrounds it; the nucleus, or center; and the **cortex**, which is made up of large fibers, running from top to bottom.

The space between the iris and cornea, called the anterior chamber, is filled with a clear solution called the **aqueous humor**. Behind the lens is a jellylike substance called the **vitreous humor**, which fills most of the eye's interior.

Q: **What's on the other side of the eye?**

A: Last, but certainly not least, we come to the **retina**, the delicate innermost layer of tissue that lines the eyeball and is directly connected to the brain by the optic nerve. The **choroid** is a layer of blood vessels that underlies the retina; at the extreme outer layer of the retina is the **retinal pigment epithelium (RPE)**.

At the center of the retina is a tiny area called the **macula** (Latin for "spot"). It's only about the size of a capital letter on this page, but it's absolutely critical to sight.

SCHEMATIC SECTION OF THE HUMAN EYE

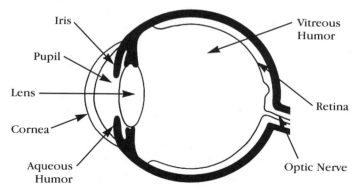

Source: American Optometric Association.

Q: Okay. Then how does the eye see?

A: The traditional analogy is to a camera, and while that's oversimplified and much used, it works. Light waves coming into the eye are bent—a process known as **refraction**—by the cornea to a point at which the image is about 60 percent focused.

The waves then pass through the pupil, which—just like the shutter of a camera—controls the amount of light that enters. The pupil becomes smaller in bright light and larger in dim light. The rays of light then enter the lens, which bends them the remaining 40 percent to focus.

Q: How does the lens do that?

A: When you're born, the lens of your eye is highly elastic. It changes shape to focus light properly, automatically getting fatter for close objects and thinner for distant objects. (In Chapter 2 we discuss what happens when the lens becomes less elastic over time.)

The shape of the lens is controlled by the **ciliary muscles**, a thin band of muscles that lines the wall of the eye. These are your eye's focusing muscles, which allow you to focus for near vision, then to refocus on objects at a distance.

Q: So now the object is completely focused. What next?

A: You've got an image focused to a sharp point on the retina—the "film" on which images are recorded. Most of the light is focused on the macula, which is responsible for "central vision"—letting you see what's directly in front of you in sharp, fine detail.

Photoreceptor cells in the retina convert light into electrical impulses that travel through several types of nerve cells and converge in the optic nerve (actually a bundle of some 1 million smaller nerves). The optic nerve transmits the image to your brain, where—extending the analogy—you "develop" the impulses into the image you see.

Q: So the macula lets me see straight ahead. What about side vision?

A: There are two types of photoreceptor cells in the retina, known because of their shapes as **cones** and **rods**. The rod cells are concentrated outside the macula, in the rest of the retina, and are required for **peripheral vision**— seeing things on the side of your **visual field** at the same time that you're looking straight ahead. They're also important for night vision.

Q: What do the cone cells do?

A: The cone cells, which are concentrated in the macula—specifically in the **fovea**, the center of the macula—are responsible for central and color vision. Each cone is filled with red, yellow or blue photopigment, a type of protein woven into the membranes of the cells. The protein is sensitive to a range of wavelengths on each side of those color peaks.

Cones need more light than rods to function well. That's why we can see colors and read far more easily in daylight.

Q: Some people seem to have a better color sense. Are their cones different?

A: There's an immense variation in the composition of cones and, accordingly, in people's color vision. While many people have some form of color blindness, as we discuss in Chapter 2, others have increased sensitivities to certain colors beyond the normal range. It's been found that nearly half of Caucasian men, for example, have a greater-than-average sensitivity to red light, and thus see reds and pinks more intensely than the general population.

Q: What controls the way I move my eyes?

A: Three pairs of eye muscles, attached to the outside of each eye, govern movement: the superior and inferior rectus (on the top and bottom of the eye); the lateral and medial rectus (on the right and left sides); and the superior and inferior oblique (surrounding the top and bottom of the eye).

When vision is normal, both eyes aim at the same spot. The brain then fuses the two pictures into a single three-dimensional image. It's this ability to see things in three dimensions, or **stereopsis**, that gives us depth perception. That's why people who lack binocular, or two-eyed, vision may be able to see clearly but lack depth perception.

Q: Anything else that makes the eye work?

A: Let's not forget about tears, that essential lubrication for the eye. Tears are secreted onto the surface of the eyeball by the **lacrimal gland**, which is located in the upper eyelid. They then drain through a small canal into the **lacrimal sac**, located under the skin on the side of the nose, and down tear ducts in the nose. That's why your nose "runs" when you cry.

But even when you're not crying, you secrete tears constantly—in lesser amounts, of course.

Q: What does the eyelid do?

A: The eyelid, which is lined with the same conjunctival membrane that covers the sclera, also serves to clean, lubricate and protect the eyeball. You might think the eyelid's shape and position are just a matter of aesthetics, but—as discussed in Chapter 2—they're also critical to how well you see.

Q: Which parts of the eye can cause problems?

A: Every part we've described is subject to disorders and diseases that can affect your comfort and vision. In the following chapters, we discuss how your vision can be affected whenever something goes wrong with any of these components.

In Chapter 2 we describe common problems that rarely lead to major vision loss. Chapter 3 is devoted to problems of the retina, which, because of the key role it plays, is of paramount importance. Chapter 4 discusses **cataract** and Chapter 5 discusses **glaucoma**, common vision problems of people over 65.

Chapter 6 covers any remaining eye issues and ways of overcoming **low vision**, the condition that's often the consequence of the eye problems described in Chapters 3, 4 and 5. The term is used by the eye care profession to describe vision that doesn't meet the needs of the individual despite the use of conventional corrective lenses. It isn't the same as blindness and can often be improved with visual devices.

Q: Does the eye serve any purpose other than seeing?

A: Yes, a very important purpose. The eye also registers light impulses that regulate the body's internal daily clock. Even people who are totally blind and can't distinguish between light and dark receive enough light to regulate their sleep-wake cycles, as long as their eyeballs remain in their sockets. For that reason, it's important to monitor eye health even of the blind.

EYE EXAMINATION

Q: What's involved in an eye exam?

A: A thorough examination includes tests for **visual acuity** (how well you can see at given distances), eye coordination, focusing ability and eye health.

Q: How is visual acuity measured?

A: With the eye chart you've probably seen all your life. It's called the **Snellen chart**, after Dutch **ophthalmologist** Herman Snellen, who developed it in the mid-1800s. When your eyes are examined, probably the first thing you'll have to do is read that chart—first with one eye covered, then the other, to test vision in each.

For each line of the chart—from 400 for the giant "E" at the top, to 20 for the fine print at the bottom—there's a number corresponding to the distance at which it can be read by a person with "normal" vision. In other words, a person with normal vision can read the line designated as "60" at a distance of 60 feet.

Q: Is that how you get 20/20?

A: That's right. For central vision, visual acuity is expressed as a pair of numbers. The first number is the testing distance, almost invariably 20 feet; the second number is the smallest line of type that the person can read at that distance.

Normal vision is 20/20. An individual who can read only down to the line designated "60" has a visual acuity of 20/60. The larger the second number, the lower your visual acuity.

Q: How large does the number have to be for someone to be considered blind?

A: When your best *corrected* central visual acuity—that is, with prescription glasses or lenses—is 20/200 or worse in your *better* eye, you are considered "legally blind" even though you may still have some vision. In fact, most people who meet the criteria for **legal blindness** retain some useful vision.

Far more people meet the eye care profession's criteria for "partially sighted"—a category that describes an individual whose better eye is between 20/60 and 20/200 even with conventional prescription lenses. States generally make 20/40 or 20/50 the cutoff for a driver's license.

People who are either legally blind or partially sighted are described by the eye care profession as having low vision. In the United States, some 4.3 million people, most of them over the age of 65, have low vision. Of these, approximately 1 million people are legally blind.

Q: Is central acuity the only measure of vision?

A: No, peripheral vision is also a factor in evaluating your vision. Normal eyes can recognize objects over an area measuring at least 140 degrees (almost half a circle). If you have a much narrower range of side vision—a condition known in the profession as "central island of vision" and, more commonly, as tunnel vision—you may have trouble walking or recognizing people in a large room, even when your central vision is excellent.

If your visual field is restricted to a 20-degree diameter (10-degree radius) or less in your better eye, regardless of acuity, you may also be considered legally blind.

Q: How is peripheral vision tested?

A: The test is described in Chapter 5, which discusses glaucoma—a condition in which an early symptom is loss of peripheral vision. We won't describe the test here because eye care practitioners don't routinely test peripheral vision unless you're over 40 or have a family history of glaucoma.

Q: What other routine eye tests are there besides the Snellen chart?

A: An eye care professional will conduct an external examination, using a small flashlight called a penlight to look at eyelids and pupils, and check the eye muscles and eye position. For example, she'll probably have you follow the penlight with both eyes while she moves it in a full circle within your visual field.

Next comes a closer look at the front parts of the eye— cornea, iris and lens—with an instrument called a **biomicro-scope**, also known as a **slit lamp**. The biomicroscope is a rather large piece of equipment on a table that's wheeled into place in front of you. It has a chin rest and a rest for your forehead, which together keep your head stationary while the professional examines your eyes.

While you stare straight ahead, your eyes can be examined

through a powerful microscope. The slit lamp also focuses a vertical beam that gives the eye care professional a view of a thin section of eye tissue.

Q: What about eyedrops? Aren't they part of an exam?

A: That's usually the next step: You'll get drops in both eyes to dilate, or enlarge, the pupils, a process that takes 20 or 30 minutes. The drops serve two purposes. They enlarge the pupil so that the inside of the eye can be examined. They also temporarily paralyze certain eye muscles to prevent the eye from focusing during the rest of the examination.

With your pupils dilated, you'll be asked again to read the Snellen chart while the practitioner tests various lenses on your eyes. To do this, she may use a **phorometer**, a device that contains hundreds of lenses that can be tried, singly or together, to determine what prescription, if any, you need to bring your visual acuity up to 20/20. She may also use a **retinoscope**, which employs a system of mirrors and lights, to evaluate your vision.

Then she will briefly reexamine you with the biomicroscope. Finally, while your pupils are still dilated, she will examine your retina with an **ophthalmoscope**, an instrument—either handheld or worn on her forehead—that gives her a clear view of the inside of your eye, including the retina and the optic nerve. Most conditions that threaten vision are sited in the retina; an important exception is glaucoma, which involves the optic nerve.

Q: And that's it?

A: Pretty much. If you wear contact lenses, your eyes will be stained and—with the lenses in place—examined under the slit lamp to ensure that the lenses fit well and have not acquired any scratches or warps.

Q: How often should I have my eyes examined?

A: The American Academy of Pediatrics recommends that infants be examined for visual deficiencies and eye muscle imbalances during the first six months of life, and that routine vision screening be included in each routine checkup. The American Academy of Ophthalmology (AAO) recommends that all children see an ophthalmologist around the time they enter kindergarten.

After that, however, the AAO says that eye examinations should be conducted only on an "as needed" basis for people under the age of 40. Between the ages of 40 and 65, people need to be examined every two years, due to the risk of glaucoma and other age-related conditions that threaten sight. After 65, an individual should be examined annually.

The main exception to those rules is the contact-lens wearer. Partly because eyes change shape and lenses may accordingly need refitting, people who wear contact lenses should be examined yearly, according to the AAO.

EYE CARE PROFESSIONALS

Q: What are the different types of eye doctors?

A: There are three main professions specializing in eye care. The ophthalmologist is the only medical doctor (M.D. or D.O.—doctor of osteopathy) with special training and skill to diagnose and treat all diseases of the eye.

An ophthalmologist has typically completed college, four years of medical school, a year of internship and at least three years of hospital-based training, or residency, in the diagnosis and medical and surgical treatment of eye disorders. Board-certified ophthalmologists have also passed an examination given by the American Board of Ophthalmology.

Some ophthalmologists complete an additional year or two of training (called a fellowship) in a subspecialty. There are nine major ophthalmic subspecialties, including retinal disorders, cataract surgery (discussed in detail in Chapters 3 and 4, respectively) and pediatric ophthalmology, or the treatment of eye problems in children.

Q: **What are the other professions?**

A: The **optometrist** is a doctor of optometry (O.D., rather than M.D. or D.O.). He is not a physician. Optometrists have completed college and four years of optometry school, where they learn to diagnose various eye disorders as well as to refract the eye—that is, determine the need for corrective lenses.

While optometrists cannot perform surgery and generally refer people with serious eye problems to ophthalmologists, in recent years optometrists' authority has been broadened. Today optometrists in all states are licensed to use pharmaceuticals to diagnose eye disease, and in most states they are also authorized to use drugs to treat eye disease.

The third specialist, the **optician**, is trained to follow the eyeglass prescription written by a doctor or optometrist, grind and formulate lenses and help fit them to the wearer. In some states such as New York, opticians can also fit and dispense contact lenses. However, opticians cannot examine eyes or prescribe corrections.

Q: **When is it appropriate to see an ophthalmologist rather than an optometrist?**

A: That depends on the condition of your eyes, your philosophy of health care and, increasingly, the rules of the insurance company or managed-care provider that covers the cost of your care.

For routine examinations and vision problems such as nearsightedness, or **myopia**, which we discuss at length in Chapter 2, you may be completely satisfied by the care provided by your optometrist. If, however, you have a disease that threatens your vision or may require surgery, you should consult an ophthalmologist.

In addition, many routine eye conditions and diseases can be diagnosed and treated by other physicians such as family practitioners. However, most lack the equipment or expertise to conduct a comprehensive eye exam or treat vision-threatening problems.

Q: But what if it's not a clear-cut decision?

A: That's where your philosophy of health care may enter into your choice of a professional. Ophthalmologists, the only eye care professionals who can perform surgery, tend to favor surgery for certain conditions, while optometrists generally support more conservative approaches such as **vision therapy**. For a discussion of these conditions and opposing treatments, see Chapter 2.

Q: What is vision therapy?

A: It's therapy based on the notion that vision is learned and that the brain can be trained to give the correct instructions to the muscles of the eye. Specialists in vision therapy—typically optometrists—offer training routines, often in conjunction with lenses, prisms and other equipment, to correct or improve specific problems such as crossed eyes in children. Therapy typically involves a session or two each week over the course of several months.

Ophthalmologists generally tend to be dismissive of vision therapy, arguing that optometrists practice it because they're precluded from more effective strategies—specifically surgery and, in some states, prescription drugs.

As that remark suggests, the debate can get pretty heated. In Chapter 2 we discuss specific applications for vision therapy, claims and counterclaims.

Q: **How does my insurance affect my choice?**

A: Health maintenance organizations (HMOs), which emphasize low-cost care, have far more optometrists on staff than higher-priced ophthalmologists, according to a 1995 study by RAND, a California research organization. So if you're a member of an HMO, you can expect to be referred to an optometrist, at least initially.

According to the American Optometric Association, optometrists already perform over two-thirds of all primary eye examinations in the United States. That percentage is likely to increase with the growth of managed care and the search for low-cost solutions.

But we're getting ahead of ourselves. Let's look now at some of the general problems that would make you seek out an eye care professional in the first place.

2 GENERAL EYE DISORDERS AND DISEASES

Q: What are the most common eye disorders?

A: The most common eye disorders are **refractive errors**, in which the shape of your eye doesn't permit it to refract, or bend, light rays properly. As a result the image you see is blurred.

If you think "refractive error" sounds arcane, think again: Myopia (nearsightedness), **hyperopia** (farsightedness), **presbyopia** (aging eyes) and **astigmatism** (distorted vision) are all different types of refractive errors.

In this chapter we describe the four types of refractive errors, as well as a variety of other disorders and diseases that commonly afflict the eye but rarely lead to low vision.

REFRACTIVE ERRORS

Q: How common are refractive errors?

A: Very. According to the National Eye Institute (NEI), which is part of the National Institutes of Health, some 120 million people in the United States have refractive errors. And most of the 25 million yearly visits to optometrists are for correction of refractive errors.

Q: Let's start with myopia. What's wrong with an eye that's myopic?

A: As you probably know, people who are myopic see well up close but have trouble with distant objects. The reason is the "length"—the front-to-back distance—of the eye.

The normal eye, as Chapter 1 explains, focuses images on the retina. The myopic eye is elongated, so images of distant objects focus in *front* of the retina, not on it.

Q: How does that happen?

A: As rays from nearby objects reach the eyes, the rays are diverging—starting from the same point of origin and traveling away from each other. When divergent rays are bent by the cornea and lens of people with myopia, they converge on the retina and the resulting images are clear.

The rays from distant objects enter the eye as parallel lines, however. When these are bent in the myopic eye, they come to a focal point in front of the retina, resulting in blurry images.

Q: When does myopia typically develop?

A: Myopia is often diagnosed in children when they are between 8 and 12 years old. It tends to get worse during the teenage years, when the body grows rapidly, and to stabilize between the ages of 20 and 40. Then, at 40, focusing on close objects typically becomes the problem.

Q: What causes myopia?

A: No one really knows, although there are two well-established risk factors for myopia. One is genetics. A study in which children were tracked for 18 years found that if both parents were myopic, nearly half the children became myopic by age 18. If only one parent was myopic, a quarter of the children were nearsighted, too. But if neither parent was myopic, only 8 percent of the children were myopic, according to the study, which was conducted by Jane Gwiazda, Ph.D., of the Children's Vision Laboratory at the New England College of Optometry, Boston.

That children inherit a myopic tendency has been underscored by other findings. In the same study, for example, many babies were found to be myopic when they were just a few months old. By age 3, all the myopic babies had normal eyesight; but beginning around ages 10 to 12, most became myopic again. (By contrast, the children with perfect eyesight at one year tended to be farsighted by age three.)

Finally, in a 1994 *Journal of the American Medical Association* article, researchers at the School of Optometry of the University of California, Berkeley, reported that even before they displayed any degree of nearsightedness, children who had two myopic parents were found to have "longer" eyes, on average, than children with only one or no myopic parent.

Q: What's the other major risk factor for myopia?

A: Remember when your mother fretted that you were straining your eyes by reading a book with small print or by sitting too close to the television? She may have had a point. Studies and national statistics indicate that close visual activity—primarily reading—significantly increases the risk of developing myopia.

While one in four American adults is myopic, for example, myopia is extremely rare in illiterate societies. In Taiwan and other Far Eastern countries where the amount of schooling has soared in recent years, the rate of myopia has also increased sharply.

Q: How does close work lead to myopia?

A: As we say in Chapter 1, the lens of the eye changes its shape through muscle contraction. The process, known as accommodation, allows the eye to bend incoming rays of light so images can focus on the retina.

Many researchers believe that hours of close work— whether it's reading, playing video games or working on a computer—disrupts **emmetropization**, the natural process by which the length of the eye adjusts so that images from distant objects remain clear.

Some researchers speculate that a defective emmetropization mechanism, or accommodation system, may be inherited. Thus it's a matter of nurture—in this case an environment that emphasizes literacy—compounding the flaws of nature. The Berkeley researchers concluded, "A particular eye size and shape may be inherited from myopic parents along with a certain level of intelligence and/or a tendency for different patterns of near-work activity."

Q: How about farsightedness? What's the difference between hyperopia and presbyopia?

A: We'll have to distinguish here between two conditions that are both widely equated with farsightedness. Technically, hyperopia, or farsightedness, is defined as a condition in which the eye is "shorter," front to back, than normal. Hence the images of close objects, like the words on this page, aren't in focus when they reach the retina.

In the case of presbyopia, on the other hand, it's the reduced elasticity of the lens that's responsible for difficulty focusing. Starting as early as age 20, the lens slowly loses its elasticity. By age 40 or so, the lens is sufficiently rigid that it cannot change shape enough to bring close objects into focus. This condition gradually worsens as people age.

While the bottom line may be the same—close objects are blurry—you can theoretically have presbyopia in combination with hyperopia or myopia, as well as astigmatism.

Q: And what's astigmatism?

A: It's a refractive error caused by a defect in the cornea, rather than a problem with the lens of the eye. While a normal cornea is smooth and round, someone with astigmatism has a comparatively oval cornea that curves more in one direction than in the other.

As a result the eye cannot focus clearly on either near or distant objects. (The word *astigmatism* is from the Greek *a*, or "without," and *stigma*, or "point.")

Corrective Methods

Q: What can I do if I have any of these conditions?

A: Eyeglasses or contact lenses are the most common methods of correcting all refractive errors. They work by compensating for the shape of your eye and refocusing light rays on the retina.

For more information about the wide array of corrective lenses, including bifocals and trifocals, see the Appendix and consult your optometrist or ophthalmologist.

Q: Aren't there glasses that correct myopia permanently?

A: You may be thinking of **orthokeratology**, in which rigid, gas-permeable contact lenses are applied in a series of sizes to alter the shape of the cornea, which results in improved vision. Some eye care professionals, generally optometrists, argue that such change can be permanent.

However, according to the American Ophthalmology Association (AOA), once the use of lenses is discontinued, the cornea returns to its original shape and myopia comes back within days. "You can't straighten a pig's tail," is the pithy analogy of Eugene Helveston, M.D., a professor of ophthalmology at the Indiana University School of Medicine, Indianapolis.

For that reason, and because surgery has become an increasingly popular and effective treatment for myopia, orthokeratology has largely been abandoned.

Q: What kind of surgery is used to correct myopia?

A: Refractive errors get refractive surgery: operations that aim to change the eye's focus by changing the contours of the cornea. The main procedure is **radial keratotomy (RK)**, an operation that was first introduced into this country from the former Soviet Union in 1978 and that is now performed on some 250,000 Americans each year. This surgery may help someone with an elongated, myopic eye, and potentially someone with astigmatism. At this point, there's no surgery to recontour the eyes of people with hyperopia or presbyopia.

Q: What happens in a radial keratotomy?

A: In this procedure an ophthalmologist makes several deep incisions, or keratotomies, around the periphery of the cornea in a radial, or spokelike, pattern. This flattens out the cornea and shortens the eye. The procedure takes less than 30 minutes and is usually performed with eyedrops to anesthetize the cornea.

A similar approach is being tried with astigmatism, with the incisions made asymmetrically to correspond to the irregular curvature of the cornea.

Q: Is keratotomy effective?

A: Yes. For people with mild-to-moderate myopia, vision typically improves within days. It's not effective for people with severe myopia.

Traditionally, however, RK has brought on a worsening in the individual's close-up vision sooner than would have been expected in the natural aging process.

For example, a recently published study sponsored by the NEI found that of 374 people who'd had radial keratotomy 10 years earlier, 70 percent of them required neither glasses nor contact lenses for distance vision. Nearsightedness had worsened for only 3 percent of patients, a deterioration easily correctable with glasses. However, 43 percent of patients experienced an overcorrection in their vision, so that they needed reading glasses.

"I think it's a safe and effective procedure, but it's important that people who want to get rid of glasses be advised about the need for reading glasses for close vision," Carl Kupfer, M.D., NEI director, told *American Health* magazine in early 1995.

Q: Can the operation be improved so there's no "overcorrection"?

A: That's currently under investigation. Clinical studies are being done now on a so-called mini-RK, a keratotomy that involves fewer cuts in the cornea (four instead of eight) and shorter incisions, with a thinner, sharper knife. It's believed that the shorter incisions, in particular, may decrease the chance of destabilizing the cornea.

But there's also a drawback to mini-RK: Shorter incisions don't flatten the cornea enough to correct all levels of near-sightedness, so it may help only the mildly myopic.

Q: Does keratotomy have any other complications?

A: While there isn't any significant evidence, there's a theoretical concern that RK may weaken the cornea, making it more vulnerable to rupture if it were to receive a direct hit.

Q: Is anything better being developed?

A: In late 1995 the Food and Drug Administration (FDA) approved the use of **photorefractive keratectomy (PRK)**, in which a laser is used to scrape a few thousandths of an inch of tissue off the surface of the cornea with high-energy, ultraviolet radiation. The procedure takes about 15 minutes, with eyedrops being used to anesthetize the cornea.

At this point, FDA approval is limited to mild-to-moderate myopia, but it's expected that individual ophthalmologists will also use it to correct more severe myopia as well as astigmatism.

Q: Is PRK more effective than RK?

A: According to the laser's manufacturer, studies of 700 eyes treated with PRK show that 75 percent of patients had their vision improve to 20/25 or better, and be-tween 3 and 7 percent had their vision deteriorate as a result of the procedure.

Q: Are there drawbacks to this procedure?

A: Studies indicate that it may take several months to bring one's vision up to par after PRK, while RK works within days. And more than 70 percent of people report some halo or glare after PRK, especially at night, in the first few months after surgery.

On the other hand, the cornea should be able to withstand injury better after PRK than after RK.

Q: Any other types of surgery for myopia?

A: Yet another surgical technique under investigation involves a so-called corneal ring. A surgeon inserts a plastic ring through a tiny incision and gently tightens it with an attached thread to flatten the cornea. The advantage of this procedure is that what's done can later be adjusted or even reversed.

In the very limited trials to date in which the ring has been implanted, it's resulted in 20/40 or better vision for most subjects, says David Schanzlin, M.D., chairman of the department of ophthalmology at St. Louis University School of Medicine, one of the two centers where the procedure is under investigation.

Q: Isn't there anything I can do to prevent myopia?

A: Not yet. But recent research is leading scientists to consider a variety of possibilities to forestall its development.

These include eyedrops that make it easier for premyopic eyes to focus on nearby objects. In her long-term study, Gwiazda found that children who would later become myopic "underaccommodated" when doing close work. Accordingly, she is now prescribing medicated eyedrops for 20 students in hopes of heading off myopia by increasing the range of accommodation.

Q: What else?

A: Another area of interest, thanks to animal studies, is a means of countering growth factors that may cause the eye to become abnormally long.

Harvard researchers have identified growth-stimulating neuropeptides that are released by the retina when vision is blurred in newborn monkeys. And several molecules that control the eye's growth have been identified in chickens, suggesting that it may be possible to prevent abnormal growth patterns that lead to myopia by using drugs that interfere with growth-stimulating molecules.

However, such drugs are many years away from development, let alone distribution.

Q: What about vision therapy? Can that be used to correct myopia?

A: Some optometrists believe it can be, although that's a minority view even within optometry. According to the AOA, vision therapy can help alleviate only borderline farsightedness or myopia.

Ophthalmologists are even more dismissive. "There is no scientific evidence that any kind of eye exercise can cure a refractive error," declares the American Academy of Ophthalmology. "A refractive error can be corrected by glasses, contact lenses or, in some cases, surgery."

However, some researchers, such as Josh Wallman, a biologist at the City University of New York, haven't completely written off the notion that eye exercises can help. "Children should be encouraged to look up from the page every so often when they are reading," he told the *New York Times*, noting that children in China are trained to do eye exercises at intervals throughout the day.

CROSSED EYES

Q: What is crossed eyes, exactly?

A: **Strabismus**, or crossed eyes, is a disorder in which the eyes are misaligned and point in different directions. One eye may look straight ahead while the other eye turns inward, outward, up or down. The misalignment may be continual or it may come and go; the turned eye may straighten at times and the straight eye may turn. The result of any of these variations may be **diplopia**, or double vision.

The two main types of strabismus are **esotropia**, in which one or both eyes turn inward; and **exotropia**, in which one or both eyes turn outward.

Q: What causes strabismus?

A: The exact cause is not fully understood, but it's clearly neurological in nature. That is, the problem lies in the brain, which controls the muscles that govern the movements of the eye.

Accordingly, strabismus is especially common among children with neurological disorders, such as cerebral palsy, Down syndrome, hydrocephalus and brain tumors. Occasionally, too, strabismus may be a symptom of a cataract in an adult.

Q: Are there any other risk factors?

A: Sometimes it runs in families, but many people with strabismus have no relatives with the problem.

Q: How common is strabismus in children?

A: Some 4 to 5 percent of all children have crossed eyes. It occurs equally in boys and girls.

Q: I thought only kids had crossed eyes, but now I've seen them in adults, too. Is this the same condition?

A: Yes. Most adults with crossed eyes have had them since childhood. However, sometimes adults develop strabismus because of certain medical problems, such as diabetes, thyroid disease, myasthenia gravis, brain tumors, stroke or other neurological disorders.

Q: At what age does strabismus usually begin?

A: Studies of newborns have found that strabismus is not present at birth but develops within the first month of life, as vision develops.

Q: Most babies look cross-eyed at least some of the time. Are they?

A: Not really. But it's true that infants' eyes drift in and out of focus during the first few months of life. Their eyes sometimes cross as they begin to focus on close objects. This is normal because the eyes typically turn ... focuses on an object.

The broad bridge of the nose and extra eyelid skin characteristic of babies add to the impression of strabismus. The confusion is so common there's even a name for it— **pseudostrabismus**, the appearance of crossed or misaligned eyes in very young children.

Children with widely set eyes and excess skin around the bridges of their noses often appear to have exotropia, in which the eyes turn outward. But usually what they have is **pseudo-exotropia**. As a child's face begins to take shape and his eyes focus better, the condition disappears.

Q: How can I tell if my child is truly cross-eyed?

A: If regular crossing persists after the age of six months, you should suspect strabismus enough to have the child screened by an ophthalmologist. Other telltale signs to look out for: Your baby seems to have trouble seeing; his eyes seem to drift; he rubs them a lot; or he tilts his head at an awkward angle.

You can make a preliminary diagnosis yourself by shining a flashlight into your child's eyes. When he's looking at the light, a reflection can be seen on the front surface of the pupil. If the eyes are aligned properly, the light reflection will be in the same location in each eye.

If the child has true strabismus, the reflection will appear in a different location in each eye. In fact, sometimes parents first notice the abnormal light reflection in flash photos of their babies.

Q: Don't most kids outgrow crossed eyes?

A: No. What happens is that their brains learn to ignore the image of the misaligned eye and see only the image

. ɪne straight, better-seeing eye. However, the appearance of crossed eyes remains, as well as other problems discussed later in this chapter.

Double vision is likely to be troublesome to people who develop strabismus as adults, because the brain is already trained to receive images from both eyes and can't ignore the image from the turned eye.

Treatment for Strabismus

Q: How is strabismus treated?

A: With early intervention. There are several treatment options, but the most common is surgery. According to the NEI, some 700,000 operations are done each year for strabismus, placing it right behind cataract surgery as the most frequently performed ophthalmic procedure.

Q: What happens in surgery for strabismus?

A: An ophthalmologist makes a small incision in the tissue covering the eye, to reach the eye muscle. Depending on which way the eye is turning, he then repositions certain muscles.

To correct esotropia, he may place the inner eye muscles farther back on the eye. For exotropia, he may shorten the muscle. In either case he may operate on the straight eye, the misaligned eye or both.

Q: Any difference between surgery for children and adults?

A: When they operate on adults, ophthalmologists like to use adjustable sutures, which allow for some fine-tuning of the alignment after surgery. First, one or more muscles are repositioned with slipknot sutures. Then, usually within the next 24 hours, the muscle or muscles may be repositioned again by untying and retying the knots under eyedrop anesthesia. In many cases no adjustment is needed, and the slipknots are converted to standard knots.

This technique isn't used for children, who would be unable to tolerate the postoperative fine-tuning. However, the panel on strabismus for the National Advisory Eye Council recommended the development of anesthetic techniques to allow adjustable-suture surgery in children, with the hope of reducing the number of reoperations. No action has been taken so far in response to the recommendation.

Q: Reoperations? You mean the surgery is repeated?

A: Often it is. Even if the surgery succeeds in uncrossing a child's eyes, they may cross again. The procedure may be repeated a few times to ensure that eyes stay uncrossed.

Q: Then—bottom line—how effective is it?

A: Results are mixed, depending on who's looking at the numbers, the type of strabismus, the age at which the patient was treated and how success is defined. In some cases—particularly when the patient is older—the eyes are cosmetically uncrossed but vision remains double.

According to the American Academy of Ophthalmology, which has a bias in favor of surgery, the results are excellent for congenital esotropia, the most common type of strabismus: 85 percent of eyes are aligned with the first procedure. However, half of those patients may need a second operation before they're out of their teens.

For its part, the AOA, whose members are not licensed to perform surgery, says that surgery doesn't work: Because people aren't taught to make their eyes work together through muscle control, the eyes turn again.

Q: What's their research?

A: The AOA cites a review of 22 studies involving 1,500 people who underwent surgery for crossed eyes. The review found that one-third achieved straight eyes and normal vision; one-third achieved straight eyes but did not attain normal vision; and one-third either experienced no change in vision and appearance or were worse after surgery than they were before.

Still, that review was limited to exotropia and was conducted 10 years ago, so the studies it examined are now 20 to 30 years old.

Q: Is there a neutral third-party view on surgery?

A: The National Advisory Eye Council's panel on strabismus acknowledges the value of surgery and notes that several advances in surgical techniques might lead to improved results and lower risks.

At the same time, the panel urges more study of drug therapy as an alternative to surgery.

Q: What's the drug therapy?

A: The eye muscle can be injected with botulinum toxin-A (Botox, made by Allergan) to temporarily paralyze it, allowing the opposite muscle to tighten and straighten the eye. Although the effects of the drug wear off after several weeks, in some cases it may permanently correct the misalignment.

The drug has been approved by the FDA since 1990 for the treatment of strabismus in patients ages 12 and older.

Q: What about noninterventional therapies?

A: A form of vision therapy called **orthoptics** is widely used by optometrists and even ophthalmologists to treat strabismus. (Ophthalmologists, however, are more likely to use this as a supplement to surgery.)

One of the most effective orthoptic therapies for strabismus involves the use of glasses with special lenses called prisms, which stimulate the ability to move eyes in and out in tandem. The NEI's Strabismus Prism Adaptation Trial found that people with esotropia who used prisms before surgery were likely to have better results after surgery and require fewer reoperations.

Q: Can ordinary prescription glasses help?

A: Yes, if the condition is **accommodative esotropia**, a common form of strabismus that occurs in hyperopic children after the age of two. "Commonly, eyes cross when a farsighted child tries to focus on a nearby object," says Susan H. Day, M.D., a consultant in pediatric ophthalmology at California Pacific Medical Center, San Francisco.

Special glasses, sometimes known as "plus glasses," correct the hyperopia and help the eyes align. Sometimes bifocals are needed for close work.

Q: **What else might be used in orthoptics?**

A: Eye care professionals may try eye muscle exercises designed to get the individual to use both eyes. The individual may read, draw or follow a moving object with her eyes, but must do so while looking through polarizing glasses that separate the sight in the two eyes. In this way the brain cannot rely on one eye alone but must practice using them both.

Q: **Are these exercises effective?**

A: Again, that depends on whom you ask. AOA studies indicate that 75 percent of people who underwent vision therapy for crossed eyes attained normal binocular vision, and 86 percent achieved the appearance of straight eyes. (The difference represents people who, despite cosmetic improvement, continued to have double vision.) Another study found that those results lasted for at least a few years.

Ophthalmologists generally limit endorsement of these exercises to cases of very small deviations such as **convergence insufficiency**, in which the eyes are misaligned only for close work or reading.

AMBLYOPIA ("LAZY EYE")

Q: What happens if you don't correct crossed eyes?

A: Half of the children with strabismus get **amblyopia**, better-known as *lazy eye*. It's a condition in which one eye has reduced central vision.

With, in effect, only one strong eye, a person with amblyopia lacks **stereoscopic vision**—the ability to see in true three-dimensional depth. Peripheral vision is unaffected, however, which may account for the medical curiosity that Babe Ruth, the baseball great, had severe amblyopia in his left eye.

Q: Is strabismus the only cause of amblyopia?

A: No, sometimes it's caused by a large difference in the degree of nearsightedness or farsightedness between the two eyes, or by a moderately high astigmatism in one eye. Amblyopia can begin developing soon after birth.

Q: How can I tell if someone has it?

A: You can't tell from the person's appearance. And, in fact, many people with amblyopia are unaware there's a problem because their brains have learned to accommodate the fact that they have only one good eye. Sometimes people learn they have amblyopia only when vision in the good eye deteriorates and they're forced to rely on their lazy eye.

With routine vision screening, however, amblyopia—or, more specifically, a discrepancy in visual acuity between eyes—may be detected in children ages three and up. In younger children it's difficult to detect a discrepancy unless it's severe.

Q: Can amblyopia be treated?

A: Yes, if—like strabismus—it's caught early. According to the National Advisory Eye Council, "in principle, at least, amblyopia is completely preventable when detected promptly." If your family has a history of lazy eye or you have other reasons for concern, you should have your child's eyes examined by age six months and annually up to age eight years, according to the American Optometric Association.

The older the child when diagnosed, the harder the problem is to correct. Many physicians say it's untreatable after age six. Optometrists, as usual, disagree, maintaining that the right mix of vision therapies can stimulate lazy eyes even in adults.

Q: How is the condition treated?

A: The most traditional approach, by both ophthalmologists and optometrists, is to cover the stronger eye with a patch, thus forcing the weaker eye to strengthen and improve vision. If this is done early enough, ophthalmologists say, it's generally successful.

If a child resists patching, his eye care professional may try glasses, contact lenses or prisms. Alternatively, she may apply eyedrops or ointments to the stronger eye, to blur its focus and force the child to put his lazy eye to work.

Q: What about vision therapy?

A: Definitely works, in the view of the AOA.
The AOA, which disputes the long-term efficacy of patching alone, believes that eye muscle exercises are critical. The first task is to teach someone to use the central part of vision in the lazy eye. Once central vision is restored, other

vision tasks are prescribed to improve eye movement, eye coordination and focusing ability.

These tasks should be done either alone or in conjunction with patching and various lenses. Between treatment sessions, for example, the lazy eye may be patched to keep it from relapsing.

Q: Do these exercises work?

A: According to the AOA, they're highly effective, even for older people. A review of published studies, mostly in optometric journals, found that success rates at all ages under 16 were quite similar. In people over 16, success was significantly lower but still approached 50 percent.

Ophthalmologists, for their part, maintain that eye exercises are ineffective—and, even if they worked, would require that the child be sufficiently mature to understand how to do them and have the patience to repeat them many times. That's rare before age six or so—by which time, they say, it's too late to correct amblyopia.

FLOATERS AND FLASHES

Q: Sometimes I see a bit of black "fuzz" in the sky or on the page of a book I'm reading. What's that?

A: It's probably a **floater**, a tiny clump of gel or cellular debris within the vitreous humor, the jellylike fluid that fills the inside cavity of the eye. Although floaters appear to be in front of your eye, they're actually floating in that vitreous material, casting their shadows on your retina.

Q: What causes floaters?

A: Generally starting in middle age, the vitreous gel begins to degenerate, forming the microscopic clumps or strands that are floaters. This is a natural process for which there's no treatment.

Floaters are also common in nearsighted people and in people who have undergone cataract operations or surgery using a yttrium aluminum garnet laser, which produces invisible infrared light. Both procedures are discussed in Chapter 4.

Q: Are floaters serious?

A: Usually they're merely annoying, not serious. For example, they may interfere with clear vision, often when you're reading.

However, your brain learns to compensate for them so that eventually, although they never go away, you rarely notice them. Until that happens, you can move them temporarily from your line of vision by moving your eyes back and forth and up and down. This creates currents within the vitreous humor that push the floaters to the periphery.

Q: But sometimes floaters are more serious?

A: Occasionally the degenerating vitreous gel may pull away, tearing the retina. This causes a small amount of bleeding in the eye that which may appear as a group of new floaters. Typically these floaters are much more conspicuous— larger and in your direct line of vision—than standard floaters.

As we discuss in Chapter 3, a **torn retina** can be serious if it develops into a retinal detachment. For that reason any sudden onset of many new floaters should be evaluated promptly by an eye care professional.

Q: What causes the flashes of light I see sometimes?

A: Sometimes, when the vitreous gel rubs or pulls on the retina, you see flashing lights or lightning streaks. (You get the same sensation when you're hit in the eye and see "stars.") The flashes may appear on and off for several weeks or months as we grow older and, unless there are other symptoms, aren't a cause for concern. However, if the flashes are persistent and are accompanied by a number of new floaters or by a partial loss or shadowing of side vision, they could indicate a torn retina. In that case you should seek immediate professional eye care.

Q: Sometimes I get a bad headache with flashing lights. What's that?

A: If the lights take the shape of jagged lines, last 10 to 20 minutes and are in both eyes, they're probably symptoms of an ocular migraine, a severe headache. Because the pain often travels to the eyes, headaches are often blamed on eye problems; but they're rarely caused by them.

INFECTIONS AND INFLAMMATIONS

Q: Isn't there a children's eye disease called pinkeye?

A: You're probably referring to **conjunctivitis**, an inflammation of the conjunctiva, which is the most

common cause of eyes looking pink or red. It's not limited to
children, by any means. Because young children tend to be
careless about hygiene, however, they're more likely than adults
to give and catch the contagious type of conjunctivitis.

Q: What is it, exactly?

A: As we said, it's an inflammation or irritation of the
conjunctiva, the thin membrane that covers much of
the eye. If you look at this membrane closely, you can see that
it's filled with fine blood vessels. In conjunctivitis the blood
vessels become enlarged and much more prominent, so the
eye looks pink or red.

Q: What causes conjunctivitis?

A: The most common causes are infection, allergies such
as hay fever, and environmental irritants such as ciga-
rette smoke, smog and chemicals like the chlorine in swimming
pools. Fatigue, eyestrain, dry air and too much sun can also
make eyes red.

There's also a type of conjunctivitis that occurs in newborns. It's acquired during passage through the birth canal of
mothers infected with gonorrhea.

Q: Apart from red eyes, what are the symptoms of conjunctivitis?

A: That depends on what's causing it. If it's allergic
conjunctivitis, your eyes may have discharge or be
itchy as well as red.

Bacterial infections usually produce a large amount of pus,
although some may produce nothing more than a mild crusting
of the eyelashes in the morning. These tend to be staphylo-

coccus or streptococcus infections, transmitted by casual contact, water or air.

Viral conjunctivitis, by contrast, usually produces a watery discharge. It's far more common, often a by-product of the common cold.

Because newborns usually don't have tears for their first few weeks, any discharge may indicate conjunctivitis.

Q: Isn't conjunctivitis highly contagious?

A: The conjunctivitis caused by bacteria and viruses is contagious—particularly the viral kind, which often breaks out among young children who play together.

To check its spread, don't share towels or washcloths, and use only disposable tissues, which you should flush down the toilet after using. If you can't avoid touching eyes that are infected—your own or your children's—wash your hands immediately afterward. Because they're more likely to spread infection, children should be kept out of school and away from other children until their infections clear.

Q: Is conjunctivitis serious?

A: In most cases it's only uncomfortable. But if there's a lot of discharge, you may have an acute infection that can damage the cornea and even cause a permanent loss of sight if untreated.

Q: How is it treated?

A: If the redness is caused by an irritant such as chlorinated pool water, it usually clears on its own or with the help of soothing, nonprescription eyedrops. If there's a possibility that it's a bacterial infection, a practitioner may give you an antibiotic ointment or drops.

There is no specific treatment for viral conjunctivitis. Many doctors prescribe topical steroids to relieve the discomfort of the condition because they decrease inflammation. Newborns with conjunctivitis must be treated promptly with penicillin, and their eyes must be irrigated with saline.

Q: Sometimes I've seen a bright red spot on someone's eye. Is that conjunctivitis?

A: It's actually a tiny hemorrhage just under the conjunctiva, and while it may look alarming, a **subconjunctival hemorrhage** is really nothing more than a bruise. A blood vessel in the eye bursts, and blood seeps between the conjunctiva and the sclera (the white, protective outer layer of the eye). The blood is gradually reabsorbed within a couple of weeks, without treatment.

It may be caused by trauma such as a blow to the eye, or by heavy lifting or straining. While anyone can get one, most at risk are people who are overweight or have high blood pressure, diabetes, anemia or atherosclerosis (the most prevalent form of arteriosclerosis, or hardening of the arteries).

Q: Are there any other common eye infections?

A: There are two other garden-variety types of infections that, like conjunctivitis, are particularly common in school-aged children.

The first is **blepharitis**, an inflammation of the eyelids caused by bacteria in the skin at the base of the eyelashes. Blepharitis tends to occur, often beginning in early childhood, in people who have oily skin, dandruff or dry eyes.

People with blepharitis develop yellowish crusts at the base of the eyelids, and sometimes small gray flakes that resemble dandruff. The scales may be itchy or more irritating, and some people develop an allergic reaction that leads to more serious complications.

Generally, though, blepharitis can be controlled through daily cleansing with warm water and a mild baby shampoo or soap that doesn't sting the eyes or with a commercial eyelid cleansing solution.

Q: What's the other infection?

A: The other condition is a **sty**, which looks like a pimple located on the edge of the eyelid. A sty is often confused with a cold sore, but in fact it's caused by a bacterial— not viral—infection of one of the small glands on the edge of the eyelid. It's not contagious.

Sties tend to occur in children because their glandular secretions are more erratic, particularly during puberty, and they're less careful about keeping dirty hands out of their eyes.

Q: How is a sty treated?

A: Hot compresses generally resolve the problem in a couple of days. If the sty persists, it may have to be surgically incised and drained, but that's extremely rare.

Q: You said conjunctivitis can infect the cornea. Can the cornea be affected in other ways?

A: Yes, the cornea can become damaged in a number of ways that leave it vulnerable to infections. Its surface can be broken by some direct injury, such as a foreign object lodging in the cornea, an abrasion from a fingernail or a nick from a scratched contact lens. Corneas also become infected after they're burned, usually by an ultraviolet sunlamp.

Corneal infections often develop in people who wear soft

contact lenses overnight. According to a 1991 review article in the *New England Journal of Medicine*, the wearing of contact lenses and the use of homemade saline solution—a common lens-cleaning solution—are two important risk factors for a chronic corneal infection.

Q: What are the symptoms?

A: Unlike many far more serious eye disorders, discussed in the following chapters, corneal infections can be acutely painful. In fact, they tend to cause pain or a scratchy feeling with every blink, as the eyelid moves over the irritated cornea. The eye also is teary, reddened and sensitive to light.

Q: But they're not serious?

A: They have the potential to be serious if they're ignored. Some infections can produce scarring and result in tissue death if untreated. "Infection of the cornea is one of the most serious conditions encountered in ophthalmology," Jay H. Krachmer, M.D., and David A. Palay, M.D., ophthalmologists at the University of Iowa, Iowa City, wrote in a 1991 article on corneal disease in the *New England Journal of Medicine*.

Q: What's the most serious corneal infection?

A: That's **herpetic keratitis**, which is caused by the herpes simplex virus type I (HSV type I), the virus often responsible for cold sores. About 500,000 cases of herpetic keratitis caused by HSV are reported each year in the United States.

Unlike most corneal infections, infection from HSV type I is contagious. (But, unlike HSV type II, which doesn't involve the eye, it's not sexually transmitted.) Yet another herpes virus—varicella zoster, the virus responsible for shingles—can also infect the cornea.

In developing countries the main cause of corneal infection is chlamydia, a microorganism best known in the United States as a cause of sexually transmitted disease. In poorer countries chlamydia often leads to a very serious corneal infection called **trachoma**.

Q: What's the herpes simplex infection like?

A: Like other corneal infections, it's painful. But it varies in duration and severity, depending on the strain of the virus. Most people have a single episode, but one in four is likely to have a recurrence within two years. If you've had more than one attack, the chances are high that it will recur.

Untreated, the process may go deeper into the cornea and cause permanent scarring or inflammation inside the eye. It may also lead to chronic corneal ulcers—small, craterlike lesions that are sometimes very difficult to heal. However, thanks to antiviral medications, herpes simplex infections rarely cause blindness.

Q: Is anyone particularly prone to corneal infections?

A: Corneal disease is more common in people with diabetes. For one thing, diabetes tends to reduce the amount of tears a person can produce, or it changes their composition; for another, the disease reduces the stimulus for blinking, which helps deliver tears to the cornea. This exposes the cornea to irritation and abrasion, especially for contact-lens wearers, and sets the stage for infection.

According to Lloyd M. Aiello, M.D., director of the William P. Beetham Eye Research and Treatment Unit at the Joslin

Diabetes Center, Boston, and Jerry D. Cavallerano, a staff optometrist, diabetic people who wear contact lenses need to be monitored closely.

Q: How are corneal infections treated?

A: Typically with antibiotic or antiviral eyedrops and/or ointments. Herpes simplex infections, for example, respond well to trifluridine (Viroptic, made by Glaxo Wellcome). Often, too, eye care professionals cover an affected eye with a patch to minimize further irritation while the cornea heals. Occasionally specialists scrape the surface of the cornea with a Q-tip or dull instrument.

If the herpes simplex infection is severe, it may be necessary to scrape the surface of the cornea or use other medications.

In cases of severe scarring and vision loss, a corneal transplant may be required. We discuss that procedure, along with other problems that can affect the cornea, in Chapter 6.

Q: Are there any other causes of eye inflammation or infection?

A: Several diseases that start elsewhere can ultimately infect the eye: Think of syphilis, in the old days, and Lyme disease today. Some inflammatory diseases such as rheumatoid arthritis can also spread to the eye, while others originate in the iris, sclera, uvea and even the orbit.

People with multiple sclerosis, a disease that affects many parts of the nervous system, often develop **optic neuritis**, an inflammation of the optic nerve. Optic neuritis is the most common optic-nerve disorder in young adults, particularly women.

Q: What are the symptoms?

A: Optic neuritis usually occurs suddenly. You may notice blurred vision in one or both eyes, especially after exercising or a hot bath; vision may be dim and colors appear faded; you may have pain behind your eyes, particularly when you move them.

In an examination the optic nerve will look swollen. However, if the optic neuritis is not affecting the optic nerve near the eyeball, it may not show up on an exam. Other tests for this problem include tests of color vision and side vision, and ultrasound and MRI (magnetic resonance imaging) scans.

Q: How is it treated?

A: Most people recover normal vision without any treatment. Sometimes ophthalmologists prescribe high intravenous doses of corticosteroids to restore vision more rapidly and, if the person has multiple sclerosis, to delay other neurological symptoms.

STRUCTURAL EYELID PROBLEMS

Q: Apart from infection, what else can go wrong with the eyelid?

A: Far more than you'd think, and often with the potential to affect your vision.

One condition, which may be present at birth or develop with age, is **ptosis**, in which the upper eyelid droops over the eye. The lid may droop only slightly, or it may cover the pupil entirely, blocking normal vision.

When ptosis occurs in children, it's usually because the **levator**, the muscle that lifts the eyelid, isn't sufficiently developed. Adults may develop ptosis with age, after cataract surgery or other eye surgery, or as a complication of other disorders such as diabetes, an eye tumor or a stroke.

Q: Is it serious?

A: In adults it's primarily a cosmetic problem, although severe ptosis can significantly restrict vision.

Children who have fairly severe ptosis that's untreated can develop lasting vision problems, notably amblyopia (lazy eye). That's because ptosis blocks the vision in one eye and also tends to change the optics of the eye, causing astigmatism. Ptosis can conceal other problems such as misalignments or crossed eyes, with the result they'll be overlooked.

Also, because children try to compensate for a drooping lid by tipping their heads back to peer underneath, they may eventually develop deformities in the head and neck.

Q: How is ptosis treated?

A: Ophthalmologists generally recommend surgery before an affected child heads off to kindergarten. The operation involves tightening the levator or, if it's extremely weak, attaching or suspending the lid from under the eyebrow so the forehead muscles can do the lifting.

For adults who have relatively mild cases of ptosis, it may be enough to take a small tuck in the levator and eyelid.

Q: Are there other eyelid conditions requiring surgery?

A: Yes. Usually they come with aging and may be treated with eyelid plastic surgery, in which the skin and muscles are tightened.

One such condition is excess eyelid skin. Eyelid skin is the thinnest skin of the body, so it stretches easily. When someone's upper lid stretches, she's often described as "heavy-lidded"; when it's the lower eyelid, it's said she has "bags." Either way, she looks tired and perhaps older than her age.

Q: Isn't that a purely cosmetic problem?

A: Not necessarily. In the upper eyelid, this stretched skin may limit the field of vision. In the lower eyelid, stretching may allow the eyelid to droop downward and turn out. This condition, known as **ectropion**, can cause dryness of the eyes, excessive tearing, redness and sensitivity to light and wind.

Q: Doesn't the lid sometimes turn inward, instead?

A: Yes, in a condition called **entropion**, which also typically occurs in the elderly. When the eyelid turns inward, the eyelashes and skin rub against the eye. Inward- or outward-turning, the effect is the same: an eye that's red, irritated and sensitive to light and wind. If entropion is not treated, an eye ulcer may form.

Q: The eyelid operations you've been discussing: Are they safe?

A: According to the American Academy of Ophthal-mology, the risk of losing vision from eyelid plastic surgery is less than 1 in 5,000 surgeries, and serious complications are rare.

However, immediately after eyelid surgery, people often have difficulty closing their eyes completely and need to lubricate them with drops or ointment. While the condition is usually temporary, there are cases in which it becomes permanent. If that happens to you, you'll have to live with **dry eye**—a condition described in the following section—or have corrective surgery.

Another cautionary note: Because postoperative skin ages and slackens badly, you may find yourself repeating eyelid surgery in 5 to 10 years.

EXCESSIVE TEARS AND DRY EYES

Q: Some people seem to be tearing constantly. Is that due to infection?

A: No, although it can easily lead to chronic infection if it's neglected.

Excessive tears, or overflow tearing, may be caused by a number of factors. In babies the likeliest cause is the presence of a membrane that blocks the lower end of the tear duct inside the nose. Normally this membrane stretches or pops open at or before birth, but in many infants it's still closed at birth, clogging the tear-drainage system.

Some 6 percent of newborns—as well as an occasional adult—have this condition, known as **dacryostenosis**.

Q: How is it treated?

A: Most tear blockages open spontaneously in an infant's first six months. In the meantime, to keep the eye free of infection, the child's pediatrician may recommend antibiotic eyedrops or ointment, along with massage twice a day of the lacrimal sac, where tears collect, to empty it of old fluids.

If there's still excessive tearing when the child is a year old, it may be necessary for an ophthalmologist to open the tear ducts by probing and irrigation. A thin, blunt metal wire is gently passed through the tear-drainage system to open any obstruction.

Q: Is that effective?

A: It usually works on small children. Adults who have this problem, however, may be more resistant to probing and irrigation, and may require the placement of plastic or silicone tubes in the drainage canals.

Occasionally a procedure known as a **dacryocysto-rhinostomy** may be needed to bypass the blocked tear duct and create a new opening through the bone into the nose.

Q: What else causes excess tearing in adults?

A: In addition to dacryostenosis, causes may include entropion, faulty blinking, orbital injury, infections of the lacrimal sac into which the tears drain and complications of burns or radiation therapy.

But the most common causes are environmental: Wind, smoke, fumes, pollen and chemical irritants can all lead to excess tear production. In addition, excess tearing usually occurs together with eye irritation in a condition called **ocular surface disease**, which may afflict people with arthritis.

Q: How do I know what's behind my excessive tearing?

A: Your ophthalmologist or optometrist may try to trace the problem by irrigating fluid through the tear-drainage system and into the nose, perhaps with the use of **fluorescein**, a nontoxic dye that glows green in purple light. He may also measure tear production or recover tears from the nose.

Q: How is the condition treated?

A: That depends on the cause. It could be eyelid surgery, if the eyelid is causing the problem, or it could be surgery to open or bypass a blockage in the drainage system. Or if the eyes are tearing because they're continually irritated or dry, eyedrops or artificial tears may help.

Q: You mean some people have excess tear problems because their eyes are dry?

A: Yes. It may seem illogical, but an eye that's too dry becomes irritated and produces additional tears, which causes episodes of overflow tearing.

Normally the eye produces tears at a slow, steady rate that's responsible for necessary eye lubrication. Dry eye is the name of a condition where the eye doesn't produce enough tears to be comfortable.

Q: What causes dry eye?

A: For some people, dry eye comes on with aging. That's particularly true for women with reduced estrogen production, even if they're not yet menopausal.

Dry eye can also result from a variety of common medications that reduce tear secretion. These include diuretics, beta blockers, antihistamines, sleeping pills, pain relievers and antidepressants. And the condition may be brought on or exacerbated by living in a dry climate with lots of wind and dust.

There's also a type of dry eye, known as **Sjögren's syndrome**, that's associated with arthritis, a drying of mucous membranes and a dry mouth.

Q: How is dry eye diagnosed?

A: It's usually self-evident. Your eyes will feel irritated, scratchy, dry and uncomfortable, or like they're burning. In some cases, however, you may have blurred vision or a feeling that there's something in your eye.

Dry eye can be confirmed with a routine eye examination, but your health-care professional may also conduct tests to measure tear production. One test, called the Schirmer tear test, involves placing filter-paper strips under the lower eyelids to measure the rate of tear production under various conditions. Or, like excess tearing, dry eye may be diagnosed with fluorescein.

Q: Is it serious?

A: It can be, if untreated, because tears play a major role in safeguarding the cornea and conjunctiva from infection and injury. Less ominous but still noteworthy, dry eye may make it difficult to wear contact lenses.

Q: Can dry eye be treated?

A: Yes, there are a number of ways to keep the eyes lubricated. If you're a menopausal woman with dry eye, your condition may well be improved by hormone replacement. But if you're not using hormone replacement, you may prefer artificial tears—nonprescription eyedrops that resemble natural tears—or another eye solution. These should be preservative-free, so as not to further irritate dry eyes.

If environmental factors are the problem, you can take any number of precautions—wear sunglasses, use a room humidifier, avoid smoking and wind—as well as use artificial tears.

Q: What if I still can't get rid of the problem?

A: If the problem is particularly severe, there are a few other options. Some people have been helped by solid artificial-tear inserts—gelatinous pellets, placed inside the lower lid each day, that release lubrication at a steady rate.

Conserving your own tears is another means of keeping your eyes moist. An ophthalmologist can close the **puncta**, or small holes in the upper and lower lids near the nose, through which tears drain. This can be done with a silicone plug or a reversible solution, or through cauterization.

OTHER EYE DISORDERS

Q: What causes color blindness?

A: Color blindness has been traced to abnormal photo-pigment in the cones, those retinal cells that—as noted

in Chapter 1—are responsible for central and color vision. It occurs when some of the pigment in one or more types of cone is missing, or the pigment is abnormal, or those cones that have pigment do not work as well as others. It's rare for all the pigment of any single cone type to be absent.

As to why that occurs, it's been long suspected—and recently confirmed—that it arises from mutations in the photopigment genes.

Q: **And the variation in pigment accounts for the different kinds of color blindness?**

A: Yes, but in most cases only one type of cone is affected, leading to a red-green deficit. People with this problem have difficulty distinguishing between red and green.

Q: **Who's at risk for color blindness?**

A: Color blindness is an inherited condition that's present at birth and far more common in men than in women. About 1 in 12 males in Europe and North America has some form of color blindness, but only 1 in 200 females has it.

Q: **Can it be treated?**

A: There's no treatment for color blindness, but people who have grown up with the condition usually adjust readily and perceive colors from other clues such as the position of lights in a traffic light. As common vision problems go, color blindness is far less disabling than many others—poor night vision, for example.

Q: Night vision? You mean some people can't see at night?

A: Many people who score 20/20 in daylight can't see nearly that well in dim light, while others have trouble with contrasts or glare—two other components of vision that are particularly crucial for seeing in dim light.

The first case involves a condition called **night myopia**, which—curiously enough—is limited mainly to young adults. The other vision problems typically afflict older people.

Q: What causes night myopia?

A: A spasm of one of the ciliary muscles that alter the shape of the lens. In some people this muscle contracts under dim light conditions, causing the lens to elongate and become myopic.

Because an aging lens is stiffer and less vulnerable to the tugging created by the ciliary-muscle spasm, night myopia is rare in old people. No one knows for sure how common it is in the young. However, Thomas Fejer, M.D., an ophthalmologist in Toronto, found that among 300 research subjects, more than one-third between the ages of 15 and 25 experienced night myopia that reduced their perfect vision to 20/40 or worse, and 21 percent tested at a dismal 20/65—well below the cutoff for corrected vision for a driver's license.

Q: Is there any treatment?

A: Yes—simply wear corrective lenses at night to bring visual acuity to acceptable levels. Unfortunately, many younger people are unaware that they may need to make such adjustments.

Q: So older people are safer drivers at night?

A: Probably not, because aging brings other problems. In fact, most people lose half their night vision every 15 years, according to Herschel Leibowitz, Ph.D., retired Evan Pugh Professor of Psychology at Pennsylvania State University.

One problem area is **contrast sensitivity**, the ability to discern an object from its background. This falls off precipitously with age.

Perhaps a greater problem is glare from headlights and street lamps. By middle age the eye's lens is scratched and the vitreous humor is packed with tiny pieces of cellular debris. These imperfections partially bend the light from headlights and street lamps, resulting in a hazy glow around objects at night.

Glasses with an antireflective coating may provide some temporary relief. For additional discussion of causes of glare and remedies, see Chapter 4.

Q: Are these problems the same as night blindness?

A: No. We're talking here about seeing poorly in the dark, not about true night blindness. The latter is a symptom of a number of retinal disorders, notably **retinitis pigmentosa**. For more information about these disorders, see Chapter 3.

Q: Sometimes I see a little yellowish bump on the white of someone's eye. Is that a tumor?

A: It's a **pinguecula**, and while it may look like a tumor, it's actually an alteration of normal tissue resulting in a deposit of protein and fat, usually on the side of the iris closer to the nose. It may also be a response to chronic eye irritation or sunlight.

Q: How is it treated?

A: It doesn't grow or threaten vision, so it doesn't have to be treated unless it becomes inflamed. It can be surgically removed, but the postoperative scar may be as unattractive as the pinguecula.

Q: What if it's growing into the iris?

A: That's an altogether different disorder, known as a **pterygium**—a fleshy growth that results from the conjunctiva growing into the cornea, usually from the inner corner of the eye.

It's not clear what causes a pterygium, but it occurs most often in people who spend a lot of time outdoors, especially in sunny climates. Ultraviolet rays and chronic eye irritation from dry, dusty conditions seem to be major factors.

Q: Does it need treatment?

A: It may become inflamed, in which case it can be treated with eyedrops or ointments. Unlike a pinguecula, a pterygium can grow large enough to interfere with vision or be quite disfiguring, and can be surgically removed. However, it often returns. Surface radiation, medication and protecting eyes from ultraviolet light and dry, dusty conditions may help prevent a recurrence.

3 RETINAL DISORDERS

Q: What part of the eye is responsible for the most serious vision problems?

A: Without a doubt, the retina. In this country most cases of blindness and visual disability are caused by diseases and disorders of the retina and the choroid, the underlying layer of blood vessels that nourishes the retina.

If any part of the retina is damaged, it's very likely that some degree of vision will be lost. Furthermore, the loss will be permanent, as the retina doesn't self-heal. At birth the eyes of every individual have their full complement of at least 300 million retinal cells; the cells do not divide or regenerate after birth.

Q: What can go wrong with the retina?

A: A number of things. In this chapter we'll describe the major diseases of the retina. The most important, in terms of the number of people affected, is **macular degeneration**, the leading cause of blindness in people over 60. Other conditions include **diabetic retinopathy**, **detached** and torn retinas, retinitis pigmentosa (RP), **Usher syndrome**, **CMV (cytomegalovirus) retinitis**, which often develops in people with acquired immune deficiency syndrome (AIDS), tumors and a retinal condition that afflicts some premature babies.

Q: Since retinas don't heal, can they be transplanted?

A: No, there's no technology for retinal transplant. However, there is a retina donor program that enables scientists to learn more about retinal degeneration through the study of donated eyes.

If you have an inherited retinal degenerative disease, including RP, Usher syndrome or inherited macular degeneration, you may arrange to donate your eyes when you die, no matter what degree of vision you have (including total blindness). The program, which is administered by the Foundation for Fighting Blindness, also accepts donations from blood relatives of people who have retinal degenerative diseases.

At the time of death, the donor's family, physician or eye bank contacts the foundation. (See Informational and Mutual-Aid Groups at the back of the book.)

MACULAR DEGENERATION

Q: What is macular degeneration?

A: It's damage or breakdown of the macula, the tiny area in the center of the retina that's responsible for central vision. Macular degeneration alone doesn't result in total blindness, because peripheral vision remains, but it affects both distance and close central vision and can make some activities such as reading difficult or impossible.

Q: Who gets it?

A: Macular degeneration is part of the normal aging process. In fact, the type of macular degeneration that accounts for about 70 percent of all cases is known as **age-related macular degeneration**, or **AMD**. (You may also see it referred to as ARMD.)

It's the leading cause of new cases of blindness in people ages 65 and older. One large study found that middle-aged people have about a 2 percent risk of getting AMD, but the risk rises to nearly 30 percent after age 75.

Another type of macular degeneration develops in children. It appears to be largely genetic and is relatively rare. In addition, injury, infection or inflammation may also damage the macula.

Q: How common is AMD?

A: Very. Of the estimated 34 million people in the United States who were 65 or older in 1995, approximately 1.7 million had some visual impairment as a result of AMD, with approximately 100,000 of those people experiencing a "devastating, rapid loss of vision," the retinal diseases panel of the National Advisory Eye Council of the National Eye Institute (NEI) estimated.

The remaining 1.6 million of people 65 or older who have AMD "will inevitably become affected with slow, progressive retinal atrophy and with severe visual handicaps," the panel added. "Most may have difficulty performing routine visual tasks such as driving, reading printed material or recognizing the faces of friends."

The council noted that as the population ages, more people will lose their sight from AMD than from glaucoma and diabetic retinopathy combined.

Q: Apart from age, are there any risk factors for AMD?

A: According to the NEI, women run a higher risk than men of developing AMD; whites are much more likely than African Americans to lose vision from AMD; and smoking may increase the risk of AMD. Some surveys estimate that 15 to 20 percent of people with AMD have one or more first-degree relatives—a parent, sibling or child—who are also affected.

Still other studies have found an association between AMD and a history of hypertension (high blood pressure), cardiovascular disease, atherosclerosis (a common form of arteriosclerosis, or hardening of the arteries), hyperopia (farsightedness), light skin and eye color, and cataracts. However, the relationship of these factors to AMD has not been systematically studied.

Q: **If one of my parents has macular degeneration, what are the odds that I'll develop it?**

A: Because the condition is caused by an assortment of genes, the hereditary pattern of macular degeneration differs from family to family. Furthermore, because AMD occurs late in life, it's difficult to determine the exact role of genetics.

To establish the pattern of disease in your own family, consult a genetic counselor or eye care professional who specializes in hereditary retinal degenerations.

Q: **Exactly what happens in AMD?**

A: That depends on the type of AMD. There are two types: **dry AMD** and **wet AMD**, so-called because of the absence or presence of leaky new blood vessels.

About 90 to 95 percent of AMD is dry. It's characterized by the slow breakdown and death of the layer of light-sensing, or photoreceptor, cells in the macula. Some research suggests that this may be related to the buildup of **drusen** beneath the macula. Drusen, which contains complex lipids (fats) and calcium, usually begins accumulating after the age of 40. However, many people have drusen in both eyes and still maintain unimpaired vision.

Q: What about the remaining 5 to 10 percent of AMD cases?

A: Those involve wet or **neovascular AMD**, in which abnormal new blood vessels grow beneath the macula, in the thin layer of tissue called the choroid. No one knows precisely why this happens, either.

One theory is that oxygen, interacting with light, creates chemical "debris" in the macula. Over time, these substances collect between the retinal pigment epithelium (RPE)—the extreme outer layer of the retina—and a thin film underneath called **Bruch's membrane**. Sometimes new blood vessels form, perhaps to clear away the debris. Because these vessels tend to be very fragile, they often leak blood and fluid under the macula.

Q: Which type of AMD is worse?

A: The wet variety, because the leaking blood vessels cause scarring and rapid macular damage that can lead to the loss of central vision in a short period of time. Although wet AMD accounts for a relatively small percentage of cases, it is responsible for 90 percent of all blindness from AMD.

Q: What are the symptoms of AMD?

A: The most common early sign of dry AMD is blurred vision, particularly in dim light. With wet AMD straight lines appear crooked because fluid from the leaking blood vessels gathers and lifts the macula, distorting vision. In both cases a small blind spot may form permanently in the middle of one's field of vision.

Both types of AMD are painless.

Q: How is it diagnosed?

A: There are several tests an eye care professional can administer that may detect macular degeneration before you're aware of it:

- Your macula can be examined for damage through an ophthalmoscope, which gives a clear view of the inside of the eye.

- You may be shown an **Amsler grid**, which is similar to graph paper but has a dot in the center, and asked whether you see wavy lines or blind spots in your central vision. All people with AMD develop blind spots, while the wavy lines are characteristic of wet AMD.

- You may be given a fluorescein angiogram to detect abnormal blood vessels under the retina. In this procedure a fluorescent dye is injected into your arm, and your retina is photographed as the dye passes through the blood vessels at the back of the eye. The dye isn't radioactive, so no x-rays are involved.

Q: Can macular degeneration be treated?

A: There's no treatment for dry AMD, but fortunately, it takes many years to impair vision seriously.

Wet AMD, which is far more destructive, may be stopped with the use of laser surgery, but only if it's caught in the first few weeks after onset. This treatment, which is known as **photocoagulation** and may be performed on an outpatient basis, involves aiming a laser light onto the back of the eye, sealing off leaking membranes and destroying new blood vessels through concentrated heat.

However, according to the retinal diseases panel of the NEI, this procedure can be used for only about 25 percent of people at risk of going blind from wet AMD. Those who are leaking blood through the fovea, or center of the macula, for example, cannot be helped by lasers.

Q: Is the procedure effective?

A: So-so. In about half the cases, the laser leaves a scar that creates a big blind spot, but it does stop the creation of new blood vessels. In the other half of cases, according to the panel, it only delays the disease's progress for a year or two, because recurrent blood vessels form on the edge of the scar left by the laser.

Q: Are there any other therapies?

A: Not yet, but researchers are investigating the possibility of transplanting healthy RPE cells into diseased maculas. At this point, however, retinal cell transplantation is still in preliminary stages in the laboratory, and scientists don't know whether the disease will eventually take over any transplanted cells.

Many scientists believe that ultimately the cure for macular and many other forms of retinal degeneration will be gene therapy, in which the DNA from healthy genes is introduced into diseased retinal cells.

Q: Can AMD be prevented?

A: Somewhat. Avoid the avoidable risks mentioned earlier, such as smoking and harsh sunlight. Wear sunglasses that block out ultraviolet rays.

And eat your spinach. That's the conclusion of a recent study conducted by investigators at the Harvard Medical School,

Cambridge, and several leading eye institutes. The study found a significantly lower risk of wet AMD among people who ate a diet rich in dark green leafy and yellow or red vegetables, and other foods high in antioxidant vitamins (A, C and E) and minerals.

The best foods, according to the researchers, were spinach and collard greens, which contained large amounts of the **carotenoids** lutein and zeaxanthin—the dominant pigments in the macula. They added that although not included in the diet questionnaire, kale, mustard greens and turnips also contain substantial amounts of lutein and zeaxanthin.

Q: Can't I just take vitamins instead?

A: Research is divided on the value of vitamin supplements in combating AMD. The Harvard researchers, for example, found no evidence that vitamin supplements reduced AMD risk.

Other studies, however, have found that people with macular degeneration improve significantly after a month on Ocuvite, an over-the-counter dietary supplement sold in the United States. David Newsome, M.D., a retinal specialist who is associated with Tulane University School of Medicine, New Orleans, and who has researched the value of supplements in fighting AMD, says his AMD patients have improved within weeks with Ocuvite Extra, which contains vitamins B and E, beta-carotene and zinc.

Q: Why is zinc included?

A: Zinc is highly concentrated in the eye, particularly in the retina and tissues surrounding the macula. Newsome says that it should be part of a broad spectrum of antioxidant dietary supplementation for anyone with AMD.

But if you try zinc, be careful of toxicity. The Recommended Dietary Allowance is 15 milligrams. Ocuvite Extra has 40 milligrams per tablet, although Newsome notes only 24 milligrams are actually absorbed by the body. He maintains that's a safe dosage.

The question of antioxidant vitamins and appropriate dosages should be more definitively answered by a macular degeneration prevention study currently sponsored by the NEI. But results won't be available until the year 2000.

Q: Any other diet advice?

A: Lower your intake of saturated fats and cholesterol-rich foods. Long-term studies of eye health and disease in Beaver Dam, Wisconsin, found that residents with the highest intake of saturated fats and cholesterol had 80 percent and 60 percent increased odds for early AMD, respectively, compared with those with the lowest intake. (You'll recall that we mentioned earlier an association between AMD and atherosclerotic disease.)

Precisely how fats and cholesterol contribute to AMD is unclear. It's possible that a presumably lower intake of fruits and vegetables—rather than the high intake of fats—accounts for higher AMD rates, conceded Julie Mares-Perlman, Ph.D., of the department of ophthalmology and visual sciences at the University of Wisconsin Medical School, Madison, in a 1995 article in *Archives of Ophthalmology*.

Q: Are there other approaches to preventing AMD?

A: Researchers from the Scripps Research Institute, San Diego, report that two proteins could block the growth of blood vessels that occurs in wet AMD (*Cell*, December 1994). Although they were looking for a means of starving cancerous

tumors, their finding holds promise as a new therapy for eye disorders like wet macular degeneration and diabetic retinopathy, in which the formation of new blood vessels in the back of the eye damages the retina. (See the section following.)

However, scientists have yet to complete toxicology studies of the two proteins—one of which is synthetic, the other genetically engineered—let alone test them on humans.

DIABETIC RETINOPATHY

Q: What is diabetic retinopathy?

A: The most common diabetic eye disease, **retinopathy** is a condition in which the blood vessels in the retina are diseased. In some people with diabetic retinopathy, retinal blood vessels may swell and leak fluid. In others abnormal new blood vessels grow on the surface of the retina. Either way, these changes may result in vision loss or blindness.

Q: Is diabetic retinopathy common?

A: It's the most common cause of vision loss in Americans 20 to 74 years of age. Each year, according to the NEI, 8,000 Americans become blind as a result of diabetic retinopathy and other diabetic eye diseases.

Q: Why do people with diabetes get this condition?

A: Diabetes is a metabolic disorder—the process of converting food into energy is called metabolism—that

results in an abnormally and persistently high concentration of sugar in the bloodstream. No one knows for sure why this should lead to retinopathy, but scientists suspect that years of carrying blood with high sugar levels eventually damages or impairs blood vessels, including those of the eye.

This faulty metabolism may also create some chemical change that makes blood vessels more vulnerable to damage.

Q: Do all people with diabetes develop retinopathy?

A: Most people with diabetes develop some degree of diabetic retinopathy during their lifetimes. And the longer an individual has diabetes, the more likely he is to get diabetic retinopathy. If you have diabetes, your risk of going blind is 25 times that of the general population.

The timing and incidence of retinopathy, however, depend on the type of diabetes.

Q: The type of diabetes? What do you mean?

A: There are two types of diabetes, and they have different risks for retinopathy.

In **type-I diabetes**, the body loses its capacity to produce insulin, a hormone that enables it to burn carbohydrates. (You may have heard type I described as insulin-dependent diabetes mellitus.) People with type I, which is generally diagnosed before the age of 20, frequently develop a mild form of retinopathy within five years of diagnosis. Eventually it becomes more severe.

Type-II diabetes is much more common, usually developing in people after age 40. In type II the body produces insulin, but the insulin does not function properly. Up to 20 percent of people with type-II diabetes already have some degree of retinopathy by the time they're first diagnosed with diabetes.

Q: But ultimately they all get retinopathy?

A: Within 10 years of a diagnosis of diabetes, half of all people with type-I diabetes and a quarter with type II have some damage to their retinas. By 20 years after onset of diabetes, nearly everyone with type-I diabetes and over 60 percent with type II have some degree of retinopathy.

Retinopathy is responsible for 80 percent of all cases of blindness among people with type-I diabetes, and for 33 percent among people with type II.

Q: So there are degrees of retinopathy? Is it a progressive disease?

A: Yes. It begins as **nonproliferative**, or **background**, **retinopathy**, which is the mild form of the disease and usually doesn't affect vision. But it may progress to **proliferative retinopathy**. The terms refer to whether or not new blood vessels are proliferating, or branching out, in and around the retina.

Q: What happens in nonproliferative retinopathy?

A: Initially, the small blood vessels in the central retina gradually narrow or weaken. Small bulges, called **microaneurysms**, develop on the vessels. Eventually a vessel may tear or break and then hemorrhage, or bleed.

If the condition progresses, the larger blood vessels may become involved. But perhaps the greatest threat at this stage is that fluid from the vessels may leak into the macula, causing it to swell and put pressure on other areas of the eye. This condition, called **macular edema**, leads to blurred vision.

Q: What exactly happens in proliferative retinopathy?

A: As we indicated, that's when new, fragile blood vessels proliferate in and around the retina at the site of previous breakages or hemorrhages. Eventually the vessels tear and leak blood into the vitreous humor, the clear, gelatinous material that fills the center of the eye. As the eye tries to repair the damage caused by hemorrhages, scar tissue forms, damaging the retina and resulting in partial loss of sight.

In some cases of advanced retinopathy, the vitreous humor—shrunken by scar formation—may pull the retina away from the back of the eye, potentially resulting in total loss of vision. (For a discussion of retinal detachment, see page 84.)

Q: Can nonproliferative retinopathy be stopped before it turns into proliferative retinopathy?

A: Yes, and early intervention is important. People with macular edema may be treated with photocoagulation, the laser procedure described earlier in this chapter. If the macula remains swollen and vision is impaired, the ophthalmologist may refocus the laser beam on unsuccessfully closed leaks—identified by fluorescein angiography—and seal individual microaneurysms.

Q: How effective is photocoagulation?

A: It got a thumbs up from the Early Treatment Diabetic Retinopathy Study (ETDRS), a study conducted at 22 clinical centers under the auspices of the NEI. The ETDRS reported that only 13 percent of eyes treated immediately after diagnosis had significantly poorer visual acuity after three years, compared with 33 percent of eyes that didn't receive the treatment.

Q: Does retinopathy always get worse?

A: Often it does, but generally the deterioration is limited. Although retinopathy is usually progressive, the advance may be so slow that vision is never impaired. Without medical intervention, however, the likelihood that an individual's vision will be impaired or lost—due to retinal detachment or extensive hemorrhaging and scarring—increases with each successive phase.

Q: Can anything be done once retinopathy reaches the advanced stage?

A: Yes. In fact, the ETDRS found that currently recommended treatments are 90 percent effective in preventing blindness in people with proliferative retinopathy.

In addition to photocoagulation, there's a more intricate and high-risk operation called **vitrectomy**. In this procedure an ophthalmologist specializing in retinal surgery removes blood and membranes, which may be blocking vision, from the vitreous humor, and cuts the scar tissue that can cause the retina to detach. The extracted vitreous body and blood are then replaced with saline, air or other gases, and occasionally with silicone oil.

Usually this procedure is combined with photocoagulation, to stop the proliferation of blood vessels.

Q: Is vitrectomy effective?

A: The Diabetic Retinopathy Vitrectomy Study reported in the late 1980s that the procedure can help maintain or recover good vision for people with very severe proliferative diabetic retinopathy, when it's done promptly—not deferred until there's retinal detachment.

Q: What are the early symptoms of diabetic retinopathy?

A: If you have diabetes, you should become concerned if your vision starts to blur or if you have light flashes or changes in color vision and contrast sensitivity—the ability to discern an object from its background.

Given the high risk for eye disease, people who are diabetic need to have regular eye checkups in which retinopathy or other conditions can be detected early. The American Diabetes Association recommends that people with type-I diabetes get a dilated eye examination annually, starting five years after the onset of diabetes. People with type-II diabetes should be examined shortly after diagnosis, and annually after that.

Q: Can diabetic retinopathy be prevented?

A: Often it can be, with good control of blood sugar levels and high blood pressure, and with a healthy diet, good eye care and no smoking.

The Diabetes Control and Complications Trial, a 10-year study that concluded in June 1993, established that tight blood sugar control prevents or delays the onset of diabetic retinopathy. The study, sponsored by the National Institute for Diabetes, Digestive and Kidney Diseases, found that intensive therapy that keeps blood sugar levels as close to normal as possible reduces damage to the eyes by 76 percent.

Q: Isn't aspirin supposed to help?

A: The ETDRS tested aspirin as a means of preventing the clumping of platelets in the small blood vessels of the retina, but found no evidence that it helped.

Q: Is there anything else that might prevent retinopathy?

A: Scientists are hoping to discover why high levels of blood glucose damage the body's blood vessels. One theory is that an enzyme called **aldose reductase**, which converts glucose into a sugar alcohol called sorbitol, may play a role in triggering diabetes complications.

For that reason researchers are looking into a class of drugs called aldose reductase inhibitors, which block the actions of the enzyme. Clinical trials are under way. But the research is purely investigational at this point.

Q: Are there any groups at higher or lower risk for developing retinopathy?

A: For no apparent reason, African Americans with diabetes are less likely than whites to develop retinopathy, even though they have a significantly higher rate of diabetes and higher diabetes-related mortality. A four-year study of 200 diabetic people, published in *Archives of Internal Medicine* in November 1994, found that the risk of retinopathy developing or progressing was 2.6 times higher in Caucasians who were diabetic than in diabetic African Americans.

Q: Aren't pregnant women with diabetes at higher risk?

A: That depends. A diabetic woman who has no retinopathy before pregnancy is unlikely to develop the condition during pregnancy.

However, the outcome is different for diabetic women who already have some retinal damage when they become pregnant. Between 5 and 12 percent of diabetic women with mild retinopathy find the condition worsens when they are pregnant.

Diabetic women who already have moderate to severe retinopathy are also at greater risk during pregnancy. In recent studies 47 percent of pregnant diabetic women had an increase in severity of retinal damage, and 5 percent who'd had non-proliferative retinopathy developed the proliferative form.

Q: What causes these rapid changes?

A: They may be due to the increased levels of hormones that accompany pregnancy. Pregnancy-induced and chronic high blood pressure are thought to play a role, too. In one study 55 percent of pregnant diabetic women who had high blood pressure in addition to retinopathy found that their retinopathy grew worse, compared with 25 percent of women who had normal blood pressure.

Q: Can a woman prevent her retinopathy from getting worse while she's pregnant?

A: Doctors have found that treating a woman's retinopathy with photocoagulation before she becomes pregnant can help reduce the risk of progression once she's pregnant.

And, like all diabetic people with retinopathy, pregnant women should get regular eye examinations to monitor the course and development of this complication. It's also advisable for women with diabetic retinopathy to be evaluated by an ophthalmologist if they're thinking about getting pregnant.

Q: You said diabetes causes other eye problems. What are they?

A: As we mentioned in the preceding chapter, corneal disease is more common in people with diabetes. Studies also show that people with diabetes are twice as likely to get cataracts as people who don't have diabetes—and to get the cataracts at an earlier age than the rest of the population.

See Chapter 4 for information about cataracts and complications with diabetes. Finally, see Chapter 5 for a discussion of diabetes and glaucoma.

TORN AND DETACHED RETINAS

Q: What's happening when a retina tears or detaches?

A: A retinal detachment is actually a separation within the retina, between the photoreceptors and the retinal pigment epithelium.

There are two main types of retinal detachments. The first, and more common, condition is better known as a retinal tear or break, in which a tear or hole in the retina allows fluid from the vitreous cavity to leak in. As the fluid passes through the tear, it may detach the retina from the back of the eye, almost like wallpaper peeling off a wall.

While it's technically accurate to define and differentiate between retinal tears and detachments, it's also something of an artificial distinction. Often there are tears as well as detachment. Or the retina tears and then detaches.

Q: How serious are these conditions?

A: Usually the tears are in the peripheral retina, where there's little effect on vision. But because such tears can lead to retinal detachment, which is sight-threatening, eye doctors often recommend surgery to repair the tears. Detachments require prompt treatment to prevent total loss of vision.

Q: First things first. Why does a retina tear?

A: As we mentioned in Chapter 2, starting in middle age your vitreous gel begins to degenerate and shrink, pulling away from its attachment to the retina. Usually it separates from the retina without causing problems. But sometimes the vitreous gel pulls hard enough—or the retina is sufficiently fragile—to tear the retina in one or more places.

Alternatively the retinal tissue can independently degenerate and tear over time.

Q: Are there any factors that increase my risk of getting a detached retina?

A: The American Academy of Ophthalmology lists several conditions that might make someone more predisposed to retinal detachment. You're at higher risk for getting a detached retina if you are nearsighted; have glaucoma, diabetes or AIDS; have a previous retinal detachment in your other eye; have a family history of retinal detachment; have weak areas in your retina that can be seen by your ophthalmologist; or have had cataract or other eye surgery, or any other eye trauma. In fact, retinas have been known to detach months or even years after trauma that resulted in scar formation involving the retina.

Q: Sounds like retinas detach pretty easily. How common is this?

A: It's been estimated that between 18,000 and 30,000 Americans develop detached retinas each year. While there are no hard numbers, retinal tears are many times more common than that.

Q: What are the symptoms?

A: Retinal tears may occur gradually and without symptoms. Sometimes, however, you may see sudden bursts of flashing lights or sparks, followed by numerous small floaters or spots in the field of vision.

If the retina actually detaches, whether it's gradual or sudden, you may have the sensation of a dark curtain falling across your visual field. If the macula detaches, your central acuity will drop abruptly, and vision may be reduced to light perception or hand movement only. These symptoms remain until the condition is corrected.

Q: How is it diagnosed?

A: An eye care professional can usually see retinal tears or detachments by looking at your retina through an ophthalmoscope while your pupils are dilated. While that's part of a routine eye exam, you shouldn't wait until then to have the condition confirmed and treated.

Q: How are retinal tears repaired?

A: There are two main surgical approaches for repairing tears: laser treatment that applies concentrated heat, and **cryotherapy**, or freezing.

In the first approach, a laser creates a tiny burn at the point of the break and "welds" the separated layers of the retina back together.

In cryotherapy a freezing probe is applied to the surface of the eye over the point of the break. The extreme cold penetrates to the retina and freezes only the area around the break. As the frozen area heals, scar tissue forms and attaches the retinal layers together at the edges of the break.

Q: Are these procedures successful?

A: Yes, as a rule. They sometimes fail, however, because membranes develop on the retina, leading to new retinal breaks and eventually to retinal detachment—which, as we noted earlier, generally requires prompt treatment to safeguard vision.

Q: Is there a different procedure when the retina is detached?

A: There are several surgical approaches, depending on the type of detachment. One procedure is known as **scleral buckling**.

In this procedure the ophthalmologist drains from the eye the fluid that's collected under the detached retina. Then she wraps a silicone band around the eye to push it slightly inward. This pushes the RPE into contact with the detached retina. Scar tissue helps reattach the layers.

The band is held in place by nylon sutures, which, though permanently in the eye, probably won't be seen or felt.

Q: What are the other procedures?

A: A relatively new procedure is **pneumatic retinopexy**, in which a pure gas bubble is injected into the vitreous space inside the eye. Because of equilibrium with body gases, the gas gradually expands, pushing the retina against the back wall.

A related procedure is the vitrectomy, mentioned in the earlier section on diabetic retinopathy. In this procedure the vitreous gel is removed from the eye and replaced with a gas bubble. Sometimes vitrectomy is combined with scleral buckling.

Q: Is it safe to have a gas bubble in the eye?

A: Yes, as long as you take certain precautions. After surgery you may have to maintain a certain head position for several days, and you may not fly in an airplane or travel up to high altitudes until you are told the bubble is gone. A rapid increase in altitude can cause a dangerous rise in eye pressure.

Q: Is gas the only material that can be used?

A: Recently the Food and Drug Administration (FDA) approved substituting a silicone oil product for gas. The oil, a clear, colorless fluid, is injected into the eye and holds the retina in place until it reattaches to the wall. Typically the oil is removed within a year after surgery, but it can be left in place in people who would otherwise require additional retinal attachment surgery.

Q: Which is better, pneumatic retinopexy or scleral buckling?

A: The procedures have similar rates of reattachment— upward of 90 percent—although sometimes a second operation may be needed to keep the retina attached.

Pneumatic retinopexy is generally preferred, because it's less invasive. A study comparing the two noted a greater chance of attaining visual acuity of 20/50 or better in people with recent macular detachment who were treated with pneumatic retinopexy.

But retinopexy isn't always an option. If the detachment is particularly severe, the surgeon will use scleral buckling.

Q: What are the complications of the procedures?

A: Pneumatic retinopexy can result in new retinal tears, macular holes and retinal folds through the macula, and the risk of cataracts from the gas bubble. Scleral buckling can also lead to cataracts, as well as glaucoma, **proliferative vitreoretinopathy (PVR)**—the development of membranes on the retina, with reopening of retinal breaks and recurrent detachment—and blindness.

Q: Are there any other procedures to repair detached retinas?

A: In sight-threatening conditions like PVR, when standard procedures aren't sufficient to reattach the retina, some ophthalmologists perform an operation called a **retinotomy**. In this procedure the physician makes a "relaxing" incision of the peripheral retina, cutting the new membranes. Essentially the peripheral retina is sacrificed in order to reattach the macula.

After the retinotomy the ophthalmologist generally also locates any retinal tears and uses laser surgery or cryotherapy to seal them. In theory the scars prevent the passage of fluid through the holes and ensure long-term reattachment. Still, the prognosis for anyone with PVR is poor.

Q: You've said that retinal detachment requires prompt treatment. How prompt, exactly?

A: Very prompt indeed—within days, if possible. The sooner the surgery, the better the chances for success.
While the NEI's retinal diseases panel concluded that "we do not understand why some patients rapidly recover visual function after retinal reattachment whereas others do not," members did note that in general, chances for recovery are

better when the retina has not been detached for very long or very far from the RPE. The panel hypothesizes that a "chronically detached, highly elevated" retina may suffer greater permanent damage from lack of oxygen and nutrients.

RETINITIS PIGMENTOSA

Q: What is retinitis pigmentosa?

A: Retinitis pigmentosa (RP) refers to a group of related diseases that tend to run in families and affect the retina, causing slow but progressive loss of vision. Specifically, photoreceptor cells in the retina stop functioning and degenerate over time.

Q: Why do the photoreceptor cells degenerate?

A: The basic cause is believed to be genetic—that is, it's programmed into your cells, not caused by injury, infection or any other external agent.

Q: How common is it?

A: RP is the most common cause of inherited blindness. It affects about 100,000 people in the United States, from all ethnic and racial backgrounds, at any given time.

It is estimated that 1 in every 80 people carries a recessive gene for RP, meaning that two copies of the mutated gene are needed to produce the disease.

Q: If I'm a carrier, how can I tell whether my children will get RP?

A: This can be complicated, because different forms of RP fall into the three standard inheritance patterns. Each type of inheritance will create a different pattern of affected and unaffected family members.

For example, about one-half of children with RP are born to parents with normal vision who carry the RP gene, while parents who have RP could have both affected and unaffected children. One type of RP affects only males; females can carry it but not be directly affected. (Nonetheless, RP occurs in men and women in roughly equal numbers.) There are also isolated cases in which one individual appears to be the only member of a family to have RP.

As with inherited macular degeneration, you should consult a genetic counselor or eye care professional who specializes in hereditary retinal degenerations.

Q: What are the symptoms of RP?

A: Symptoms vary, depending on which type of photoreceptor cell is affected most. (You'll remember that photoreceptor cells can be either cones, which are found in the macula and are responsible for central vision, or rods, which are concentrated in the rest of the retina and are required for peripheral vision.)

In a person with predominantly rod cell degeneration, night blindness and loss of peripheral vision are the most common symptoms. In people with degeneration primarily of cone cells, the initial symptoms are decreased central vision and the onset of color blindness. (While decreased central vision is also a symptom of AMD, in RP it occurs decades earlier.)

Q: How quickly does RP progress?

A: The first symptoms of retinitis pigmentosa usually occur in youth or young adulthood. Most people with RP are legally blind by the age of 40, although many retain a small amount of sight.

Usually the degeneration is gradual, although the pace may vary even from one family member to the next. Some women say their RP progressed more rapidly during pregnancy, but this issue has never been studied in a systematic way. Sometimes people with RP say they see better on one day than on another, and fatigue and emotional stress may also temporarily affect vision.

Progression of the disease, however, is unstoppable.

Q: How is it diagnosed?

A: A number of tests can be performed, preferably by a physician who specializes in the retina, to detect RP through characteristic retinal changes. Some of the tests monitor the symptoms we mentioned earlier—central and side vision, color perception, adaptation to the dark—while others take an electrophysiological measure of the retina.

Q: An electrophysiological measure? How is that done?

A: The most common test is an **electroretinogram**. First, one eye is patched, and drops and a contact lens are inserted into the other. A machine flashes bright lights at the exposed eye and makes a record—an electroretinograph—of the electrical currents that are produced in the retina. Then the second eye is patched and the first eye is tested.

In healthy photoreceptor cells, there is a characteristic intensity and speed of the electrical signal. These decline as the photoreceptors die.

Q: Is RP associated with other diseases?

A: Some 10,000 to 20,000 people who have RP also have Usher syndrome, which involves the loss of hearing as well as vision. Usher syndrome, which is also inherited, is the major cause of deaf-blindness in the world.

Q: Is it a progressive disease like RP?

A: That depends on the type of Usher syndrome. People with Usher syndrome type I are born with virtually no hearing, and in adolescence usually begin to exhibit the first signs of RP. People with type II are moderately to severely hearing-impaired at birth and remain that way throughout their lives, although they also develop RP in adolescence. In type III, which was discovered in 1995, hearing loss is progressive, starting at birth.

Q: What causes Usher syndrome?

A: Researchers believe that it's caused by mutations in certain genes that are necessary for both normal vision and normal hearing. These mutations, which are inherited, give faulty messages to the sensory retinal and inner ear cells, leading to their loss of function.

The three types of Usher syndrome appear to be caused by defects in different genes.

Q: Can RP and Usher syndrome be treated?

A: While there's no cure, recent evidence indicates that vitamin A palmitate—a form of vitamin A—may slow the progression of retinal degeneration in some people with RP or Usher syndrome.

A six-year clinical study, by researchers at Harvard Medical School, reported in 1993 that adults with RP who supplemented their diets with 15,000 international units (I.U.) of vitamin A palmitate daily had a 20 percent slower average annual decline in remaining retinal function. The study included people with several common forms of RP and Usher syndrome type II.

Based on this finding, researchers estimated that an average person who started taking a daily supplement at age 32 would retain some useful vision until age 70, while a person who didn't take the supplement would have no useful vision by age 63.

Q: Is it safe to take a lot of vitamin A?

A: There's been no toxicity reported in healthy adults taking 15,000 I.U. daily. But people taking the supplement are advised to have their liver function tested—before they begin the regimen and each year after that.

And they shouldn't take more than 15,000 I.U. "One of my biggest concerns is that people will make the mistake of thinking that vitamin A supplementation in excess of 15,000 I.U. will provide even greater benefit," says Eliot Berson, M.D., the study's principal investigator and professor of ophthalmology at Harvard. That's not true, he notes, adding that doses over 25,000 I.U. daily have been linked to liver disease.

Pregnant women are advised not to take 15,000 I.U., because of the danger of birth defects. And, because the study involved adults, there are no recommendations for people under the age of 18.

Keep in mind, too, that the study specifically tested vitamin A in palmitate form—not supplements of beta-carotene, a natural precursor of vitamin A.

Q: Are any other vitamins helpful?

A: None has been identified. But another important finding of the study was that vitamin E supplements, in daily doses of 400 I.U., actually increased the rate of retinal degeneration. Researchers recommended that people with RP avoid high-dose vitamin E supplements.

There is no evidence, however, that normal dietary amounts of vitamin E are harmful.

Q: Are there any other treatments for RP?

A: No, but a few potential therapies are under study. As we mentioned earlier, the transplantation of healthy retinal cells is under investigation. The good news is that studies have found that when photoreceptor cells are transplanted into the retinas of laboratory animals, some normal features either are maintained or develop after transplantation. This has yet to be tried, however, in animals with an RP-type degeneration.

As researchers identify more of the mutant genes that contribute to RP, gene therapy is another down-the-road possibility. Growth factors—small proteins manufactured naturally by cells to reduce cellular injury and prevent cell death—also hold some promise. Scientists have demonstrated that several different growth factors, injected into the eye, can keep injured and dying photoreceptor cells alive in rats, and can even delay an inherited degeneration.

CMV RETINITIS

Q: Earlier you mentioned that people with AIDS develop retinal problems. What are they?

A: It's very common for people with AIDS to get tiny amounts of bleeding and white spots in the retina. These white spots are called *cotton wool spots* because of the way they affect vision. They appear to be a consequence of the human immunodeficiency virus (HIV) and, in fact, are sometimes the first symptom of the disease.

These spots come and go, don't threaten vision and don't require treatment.

Q: But don't people with AIDS develop serious eye problems?

A: Yes, specifically CMV retinitis, an infection caused by the cytomegalovirus (CMV) that spreads across the retina, cell by cell. Unchecked, the virus can spread from one eye to the other and cause blindness. Or it can cause retinal detachment, which can also result in blindness.

Before the AIDS epidemic, CMV retinitis was rare. Now the NEI estimates the disease occurs in about one in four people with AIDS. Most infections occur when the number of T cells—a special kind of white blood cell—gets dangerously low, usually under 40. (People are considered to have moved from HIV-positive to AIDS when their T cells drop below 200.)

Q: But CMV retinitis can be treated?

A: Yes. Traditionally it's been treated with daily intravenous doses of one of two drugs—foscarnet (Foscavir, by Astra), which is specifically for people with AIDS, and ganciclovir (Cytovene, made by Hoffmann-La Roche), which is for all immunocompromised people, including transplant recipients. The FDA recently gave ganciclovir clearance to be marketed as a preventive treatment as well as for maintenance therapy.

Neither drug kills the virus or restores the function of previously infected areas. But it may stop or slow the spread, and if only one eye is infected, the medicine may protect the other. Even if they receive treatment, however, perhaps a quarter of the people who develop CMV retinitis still develop retinal detachment requiring surgery.

Q: Is one drug more effective than the other?

A: A study reported in the *New England Journal of Medicine* in 1992 found they were equally effective in halting the progression of CMV retinitis and in preserving vision.

However, both drugs pose significant risks for people with AIDS. Foscarnet has toxic effects, including seizures. Ganciclovir cannot generally be taken with full doses of AZT, the antiretroviral drug used to treat AIDS, because both drugs act as bone marrow suppressants. The same study found that patients treated with foscarnet lived a few months longer than those who received ganciclovir.

Drug toxicity is a particularly critical problem, since AIDS patients lack the immune system response necessary to fight the virus and must take the drugs for the rest of their lives.

Q: Doesn't sound too great. Isn't there any alternative?

A: Yes. In March 1996 the FDA approved the marketing of a capsule saturated with ganciclovir that, implanted in the eye, bathes the eye constantly with the drug. Delivering the drug to the eye rather than through the bloodstream lets the eye get a more concentrated dose and may reduce complications. When the drug is depleted, after five to eight months, the device—Vitrasert, made by Chiron—can be replaced.

Archives of Ophthalmology in 1994 reported that of 39 eyes treated with this implantation, 34 retained nearly perfect vision eight months later.

Recently, an advisory panel to the FDA approved another drug, which requires intravenous infusions every two weeks rather than daily. Still other drugs are being developed.

Q: **Are there special precautions that people with AIDS should take?**

A: Because most infections occur when the number of T cells gets dangerously low, the American Academy of Ophthalmology recommends that people who are HIV-positive be examined by their eye doctors every three months when their T-cell count falls below 250.

If you're HIV-positive, get a checkup immediately if you see vitreous floaters or flashing lights, or develop blind spots or blurred vision.

TUMORS

Q: **You mentioned earlier that tumors can affect the retina. Do you mean cancer?**

A: Tumors, cancerous or benign, can form in almost all tissues within the eye. But tumors of the retina or choroid—the underlying layer of blood vessels that nourishes the retina—are especially serious, threatening life as well as vision.

For a discussion of tumors that occur elsewhere in the eye, see Chapter 6.

Q: What types of tumors involve the choroid and retina?

A: The most common malignant tumor of the eye is **choroidal melanoma**, which arises from pigmented cells of the choroid. Usually it occurs in the middle-aged or elderly. There are more than 1,500 new cases of choroidal melanoma diagnosed each year in the United States.

Q: What are the symptoms?

A: People are typically unaware of this tumor until they begin losing vision. But it may also be discovered, as a tiny, mushroomlike growth, in the course of a routine eye examination.

Q: How is this type of tumor treated?

A: Radiation therapy and removal of the eye are both options, but there's little evidence to indicate which is more effective (or whether either works). In about half of the cases, even if the eye is removed, the tumor has spread to other parts of the body and often proves fatal. A national study is evaluating different treatment methods, but it will be many years before the results are known.

Q: Are there tumors that affect the retina?

A: **Retinoblastoma**, a genetically determined and often inherited tumor, is the most common intraocular cancer of childhood. It's typically found in children from birth to age seven, usually by the second or third year of life.

Between 300 and 400 new cases of retinoblastoma are diagnosed each year in the United States, and about 40 percent involve both eyes.

Q: Do kids survive this tumor?

A: Yes, although generally at considerable cost. The overall survival rate is about 90 percent, but often it's achieved through surgical removal of the affected eye or eyes (resulting in facial asymmetry as a complication, as the child's head is still developing). Furthermore, it's typically treated with radiation, which slightly increases the likelihood that a new, unrelated tumor will develop over the lifetime of the survivor. That's because radiation increases mutations in the DNA of normal tissues as well as in the tumor.

The good news is that surgeons are beginning to use cryotherapy, which allows them to preserve the eye and forgo radiation, too. In addition, the gene responsible for retinoblastoma has been isolated, cloned and sequenced, creating the potential for more successful treatment and prevention.

OTHER RETINAL PROBLEMS

Q: Don't some premature babies have specific eye problems?

A: Premature babies, particularly those weighing less than three pounds at birth, sometimes develop a condition called **retinopathy of prematurity (ROP)** or **retrolental fibroplasia**, in which abnormal blood vessels and scar tissue grow over the retina.

Q: What causes this condition?

A: No one knows. In the past, blame has been laid on both the fluorescent lighting used in hospital nurseries and the pure oxygen preemies receive because their lungs aren't functioning properly. Newer evidence indicates that other factors are more significant—specifically, the degree of prematurity and birth weight.

The most premature and tiniest babies have the highest odds of developing ROP. A baby weighing three pounds at birth has only a 5 percent chance of developing ROP, while a baby weighing less than two pounds has a 40 percent chance.

Unfortunately, because technology has improved the survival chances of very small babies, ROP has become more common.

Q: Is it serious?

A: In many children the condition subsides without affecting vision. In others with more extensive ROP, bleeding and scar tissue may lead to distortion or detachment of the retina. This may result in moderate to severe loss of vision. Many children with ROP are nearsighted.

Only a very small percentage of babies become blind. However, they have a higher-than-average chance of later developing complications such as glaucoma and misaligned eyes.

Q: Can ROP be treated?

A: Babies with relatively mild ROP recover without treatment. In more severe cases, ophthalmologists may use laser photocoagulation or cryotherapy—similar to that used to repair retinal tears—to slow down or reverse the abnormal growth of blood vessels and scar tissue. If severe ROP pulls the retina out of place, more complex surgery can sometimes restore limited vision.

Q: Are there any other problems in which the retina is affected?

A: People with sickle-cell anemia may develop a condition known as sickle-cell retinopathy. Sometimes this can be severe enough to cause vitreous hemorrhage or retinal detachment, threatening vision and requiring treatment with one or more of the procedures described earlier.

Q: What is sickle-cell anemia?

A: It's an inherited disease of the red blood cells, which become crescent- or sickle-shaped from oxygen deficiency. The disease, which primarily afflicts African Americans, often leads to death in childhood or adolescence from infection or stroke.

4 CATARACTS

Q: What is a cataract?

A: It's a clouding in the transparent lens of the eye that blocks or distorts light, causing loss of vision.

The lens consists mostly of water and protein. Eventually some of the protein may clump together and start to cloud a small area of the lens. That area is called an **opacity**. Over time the opacities increase in number, clouding more of the lens, until the amount of light entering the eye and striking the retina is markedly reduced.

Q: What causes cataracts?

A: In a word, age—cataracts are a normal part of aging. This process may begin in a person's 40s or 50s, but usually it isn't until someone's 60s that vision is affected. According to the U.S. Department of Health and Human Services, about half of Americans ages 65 to 74, and about 70 percent of those age 75 and over, have cataracts.

Q: So cataracts never occur in the young?

A: Rarely. Cataracts can occur in newborns with **galactosemia**, a rare disease in which babies lack an enzyme that enables them to digest galactose (a component of lactose, the principal sugar in milk). The undigested galactose is converted to a substance that accumulates in the lens and usually causes cataracts. If the condition is recognized within the infant's first month and soy milk is substituted, the cataract will disappear.

Milder forms of milk intolerance may also be one cause of the cataracts that babies and children sometimes develop.

And some babies are born with cataracts in one or both eyes. Congenital cataracts can be caused by prematurity or if the mother, during pregnancy, develops German measles or takes certain medications such as steroids.

Q: Are there different types of cataracts?

A: Yes, because the opacities initially form in different parts of the lens.

The lens has three parts: the nucleus, or center; the capsule, a thin membrane that completely surrounds the lens; and the cortex, the fibrous area in between.

Nuclear sclerosis, the most common type of opacity, describes a condition in which the nucleus gradually becomes more dense and opaque. In a **cortical cataract**, it's the outer shell of the lens that becomes progressively more opaque.

When most of the clouding is centered on the back, or posterior, surface of the lens, it's called a **posterior subcapsular (PSC) cataract**. PSC cataracts are more common in people with diabetes or who have used steroids for a long time.

Q: Do the different cataracts affect vision differently?

A: At first, vision may be affected differently based on where the opacities are concentrated. For example, you may temporarily develop double vision in the eye with a cataract if one part of the lens has more opacities than another. This condition is most common when the cataract starts in the nucleus.

If you have a PSC cataract, you'll have more trouble seeing in bright light. The reason is that on a sunny day, the pupil contracts to the size of the clouded center. For those with PSC cataracts, vision actually improves on overcast days.

However, as the opacities increase, the cataracts and vision impairment become more alike, and are treated the same.

Q: How can I tell if I'm getting cataracts?

A: The most common indication is vision that's cloudy or blurred, almost as if one were looking through water. In fact, the word *cataract* means waterfall in Latin.

Other changes also start slowly and gradually, becoming more pronounced over time. Often colors look faded or yellow. Because cataracts cause light entering the eye to be scattered, you may develop problems with glare from sunlight or light from a lamp or an oncoming car's headlights at night.

Q: Is it true that sometimes people's sight seems to improve when they get cataracts?

A: Yes. Sometimes older people who normally wear reading glasses find they're able to read without their glasses and think their eyesight is improving. In fact, it's generally an early indication that a nuclear sclerosis cataract is developing: The thicker lens creates the elongated eye characteristic of nearsightedness.

Q: How fast does a cataract develop?

A: That's all in the eyes of an individual—and may vary even within the individual's pair of eyes. As a rule, cataracts in younger people and people with diabetes progress rapidly over a few months, while cataracts in the elderly progress over a period of years.

Q: Does a person usually get a cataract in just one eye, or both?

A: Most people with cataracts have the condition in both eyes. One eye may be worse than the other, though, because cataracts all develop at different rates.

Q: How is a cataract diagnosed?

A: Generally through a routine eye exam, as described in Chapter 1. The Snellen chart gives a measure of your visual acuity. In the slit-lamp examination, the eye care professional focuses a vertical slit of light onto your cataract to see how dense the cataract is and also to determine whether your cornea is healthy enough to withstand surgery, should you decide to have the cataract removed. (This is discussed further on page 111.)

In addition, there are several tests commonly performed prior to cataract surgery. We'll discuss those and the controversy that attends some of them in the section on surgery later in this chapter.

Q: Are there any alternatives to surgery?

A: There are stopgap measures, such as different glasses for someone who is becoming nearsighted because a cataract has thickened the nucleus of the lens. If the cataract is causing glare, sometimes drops keep the pupil dilated. Magnifying glasses or other devices may also improve low vision, as described in Chapter 6.

Currently, however, there is no nonsurgical treatment for cataracts that can restore the natural lens to its clear state.

Q: Apart from aging, what causes cataracts?

A: There are a number of causes, starting with diabetes. According to a 1981 study of nearly 5,000 people in Framingham, Massachusetts, a person with diabetes under the age of 70 has a 30 to 40 percent greater chance of having a cataract than a person without diabetes. (After the age of 70, they have an equal chance.)

The reason, researchers have established, is the high blood sugar concentration that's characteristic of diabetes. The blood sugars, known as aldose sugars, dissolve into the lens of the diabetic person and are converted by the aldose reductase enzyme into substances that bloat the lens, resulting in a cataract.

You'll remember that the aldose reductase enzyme, as discussed in Chapter 3, may also contribute to diabetic retinopathy.

Q: Are there any other risk factors for cataracts?

A: Malnutrition and certain medical problems that cause malnutrition by causing low blood calcium can lead to cataracts. Of far greater concern, at least in the generally well-nourished United States, are some illnesses, such as arthritis

and asthma, that are best controlled with steroids. In some people even small amounts of steroids can result in cataracts.

People whose work exposes them to intense heat, such as glassblowers, or to electric shock, such as electricians, are also at higher risk; so, too, are people who have glaucoma in their families.

A cataract can also result from injury to the eye, whether it's surgery, a physical blow or head trauma. The ciliary muscles that surround the lens are connected to it by thousands of thin strands called **zonules**. In a trauma like a car crash, the zonules are disturbed, dislodging the lens from its normal position and sometimes causing a cataract.

Q: Isn't sunlight supposed to cause cataracts?

A: That's right. Ultraviolet light, x-rays and radiation have all been linked to cataract formation. All are sources of oxidation, a metabolic process that has been implicated as a cause of cataracts (as well as a cause of cancer and heart disease).

Studies of the incidence of cataracts show a uniformly higher incidence in sunnier parts of the United States or in countries close to the equator. And, according to a 1991 United Nations panel of scientists, the depletion of the earth's ozone layer will lead to an increase of cataracts worldwide.

In addition, one study reports that people who are treated with total-body irradiation during bone marrow transplantation are likely to develop cataracts within 10 years (*Annals of Internal Medicine*, 1993). The researchers, physicians at the University Hospitals in Basel, Switzerland, recommend that preventive measures, such as lens shielding during irradiation, be considered.

Q: So I don't have to give up drinking and smoking to avoid cataracts?

A: Wait—we just hadn't gotten around to those! In fact, alcohol and cigarettes have both been linked to a higher-than-average incidence of cataracts.

A study published in the *American Journal of Preventive Medicine* in 1994, of approximately 18,000 male doctors followed over a six-year period, found that the risk of cataracts was 30 percent greater for daily drinkers, compared with those who drank less often than once a month. The same study also found that people who smoke more than a pack of cigarettes a day have more than double the risk of developing cataracts that nonsmokers have.

Those odds were confirmed by another study, of 70,000 female nurses followed for eight years. In reviewing the results, Sheila West, M.D., an ophthalmologist at Johns Hopkins Hospital, Baltimore, concluded that 20 percent of all cataract cases in the United States could be prevented if people didn't smoke.

Q: Summing up, then: How can I help prevent cataracts?

A: As we noted earlier, don't smoke and don't drink to excess, and try to minimize use of steroids. And protect your eyes from sunlight. Wear sunglasses that screen out ultraviolet light rays or regular eyeglasses with a clear, anti-UV coating. (See the Appendix for more information about eye devices.)

Q: What about diet?

A: Just as you were told for years, carrots really are good for your eyes—at least in preventing cataracts. The nurses' study mentioned previously showed that women who had a very high intake of vitamin A in their diets had a 39 percent lower risk of developing cataracts than did women with very low levels of vitamin A in their diets.

The value of vitamin supplements is less clear. In the nurses' study, women who took antioxidant vitamin C supplements for 10 or more years reduced their risk of cataracts by 45 percent. On the other hand, the study of male physicians found that individual supplements of vitamins C and E had no effect, although multivitamin supplements may slightly reduce the risk of developing cataracts. The researchers concluded that multivitamins may contain other components that prevent cataract formation.

Q: **Are there any medications to prevent cataracts?**

A: The same study that looked at the impact of aspirin on diabetic retinopathy—mentioned in Chapter 3— found that aspirin didn't reduce the risk of developing cataracts, either.

Some preliminary studies are now looking at drugs that might be used to control or prevent cataracts, such as eyedrops that neutralize the excess hydrogen peroxide found in aqueous fluid—the watery fluid that surrounds the lens and that, many researchers believe, causes cataracts to form. This research, however, is at a purely experimental stage.

CATARACT SURGERY

Q: **Is cataract surgery common?**

A: Very. About 1.35 million Americans have cataract surgery each year, according to the National Eye

Institute (NEI). Cataract surgery is the most common surgical procedure performed on the elderly in this country.

Criteria for Surgery

Q: **I've always heard that cataracts had to be "ripe" before they could be removed. What does "ripe" mean?**

A: At one time cataracts had to have achieved a certain density, or "ripeness," before they could be removed. For the past several decades, however, improvements in surgical technique have allowed the removal of cataracts at any stage in their development, although certain minimum standards are generally agreed upon within the medical profession.

For example, surgery would never be done on an eye with a mild cataract that reduces vision merely to a level of 20/25 or 20/30, or perhaps to 20/40. Once that 20/40 threshold has been crossed, the decision to have cataract surgery depends on a variety of factors.

Q: **What factors?**

A: You'd think there would be an easy answer to that, such as "when your vision is 20/60," but—in our cost-conscious environment right now—the timing of surgery has become a contentious area. Recently the Health Care Financing Administration (HCFA), the federal agency that runs Medicare and Medicaid, proposed that eye surgeons show that the removal of a cataract is medically necessary.

"The mere presence of a cataract does not mean that surgery is needed," said Bruce C. Vladeck, head of HCFA. "Surgery will not be considered necessary if the individual is able to function normally or if the condition can be corrected with eyeglasses."

Q: Why does HCFA have a say about cataract surgery?

A: Through Medicare, HCFA spent about $1.4 billion in 1994 on cataract surgery and related procedures. A 1993 report by the federal General Accounting Office said that Medicare spent $204 million in 1991 on inappropriate cataract surgery.

At this point, however, a comparatively hard line on cataract surgery is only in the proposal stage, and may not become policy for some time yet, if it becomes policy at all.

Q: You said this was an area of contention. Who objects to the HCFA's proposal?

A: Ophthalmologists—virtually all of whom, whatever their specialties, perform cataract surgery.

The profession's view is that the vast majority of cataract operations are necessary. "The decision for cataract surgery should be based on sound medical opinion and functional impairment, and not on budget-driven health-care policies," says H. Dunbar Hoskins Jr., M.D., executive vice president of the American Academy of Ophthalmology.

Q: What's the government guideline for "medically necessary"?

A: The government recommendation follows a 1993 report by the Clinical Practice Guideline panel on cataracts, which took a comparatively go-slow approach to surgery.

The panel advised against cataract surgery solely to improve vision if: (1) the patient does not desire surgery, (2) glasses or visual aids provide satisfactory functional vision, (3) the patient's lifestyle is not compromised or *(4)* the patient is medically unfit.

The panel's report added that depending on the degree of functional impairment, patients should explore other options such as stronger eyeglasses or magnifying lenses before choosing surgery.

Q: **Aren't there any tests that establish the need for surgery?**

A: The panel said, essentially, that the tests ophthalmologists traditionally rely on to make recommendations about surgery are largely irrelevant.

Q: **What are the tests?**

A: In addition to visual acuity, the standard battery of tests includes contrast-sensitivity testing, glare testing, **potential vision testing** and **specular photographic microscopy**.

Q: **Would you go over each of these in turn?**

A: Contrast-sensitivity testing attempts to determine the eye's ability to detect subtle variations of shading by presenting letters or figures that are varied in contrast. The simplest tests employ reading cards or eye charts similar to the Snellen chart.

Glare testing may involve a variety of devices, from penlights to much more expensive measures, to quantify the degree of visual impairment caused by glare.

Tests of potential vision attempt to determine whether the person's vision loss is due primarily to cataracts or to another eye problem. The test may be conducted with a pinhole device that allows the person to read the eye chart as if the cataract were not present. Far more rare, and expensive, are electro-physiologic tests that allow the practitioner to make electronic measurements of the person's response to visual stimuli.

Specular photographic microscopy evaluates the **endo-thelium**, the innermost layer of the cornea, and counts its cells. The endothelium is critical because it keeps the cornea clear by removing fluid. Since cataract surgery usually reduces endothelial cell density, the test seeks to determine whether the cornea is strong enough to stand up to surgery.

Q: They all sound useful. What's wrong with them?

A: The Clinical Practice Guideline panel's 1993 report raised different objections to each test, but noted that in general the standard clinical examination provides enough information about the extent to which a cataract impairs vision. The experts underscored that it was up to each patient to decide when and whether vision impairment was severe enough to warrant surgery.

Q: Then if it's up to me, how can I decide whether I need surgery?

A: In 1995 the Cataract Patient Outcomes Research Team, funded by the Agency for Health Care Policy and Research, offered a new measure, the **VF-14**, which is a visual function index to measure cataract-related impairment of abilities to perform 14 everyday activities.

In tests on patients before and after surgery with correc-tive lenses, the VF-14 was found to be a better measure of patient satisfaction with their vision than several measures of visual acuity.

Q: What are the 14 activities?

A: In no particular order, they are:

1. Reading small print, such as labels on medicine bottles, a telephone book or food labels

2. Reading a newspaper or book

3. Reading a large-print book or newspaper or the numbers on a telephone

4. Recognizing people when they are close up

5. Seeing steps, stairs or curbs

6. Reading traffic, street or store signs

7. Doing fine handwork, such as sewing, knitting, crocheting or carpentry

8. Writing checks or filling out forms

9. Playing games like bingo, dominos, card games or mah-jongg

10. Taking part in sports like bowling, handball, tennis or golf

11. Cooking

12. Watching television

13. Daytime driving

14. Nighttime driving

Q: If I can still function all right with cataracts, is it safe to delay surgery?

A: Yes, in general. Allowing a cataract to grow usually doesn't hurt your eye or make surgery more difficult later. But there are exceptions.

Q: What are these exceptions?

A: If you have a cataract in one eye only, you will rely exclusively on your good eye, and the eye with a cataract may drift out of alignment—usually outward. However, unlike the crossed-eyes conditions described in Chapter 2, you may not be bothered by double vision because the cataract is blocking vision in one eye.

According to Julius Shulman, M.D., an ophthalmologist in New York City and author of *Cataracts*, in rare instances a cataract may get so big and swollen that it blocks free passage of fluid from the eye. This can lead to the onset of glaucoma, necessitating emergency cataract removal. This condition is reversible as long as the condition is treated promptly.

A cataract can also grow to the point where any further growth will make removal more difficult. Much more rarely, an extremely advanced cataract can rupture in the eye, causing considerable inflammation.

However, these are exceedingly rare situations. Long before your cataract grows that large, you'll probably take the plunge and have surgery.

Q: Let's say I've decided to have my cataract removed. Are there any other preoperative tests that are useful?

A: Yes. Cataract surgery involves not only extraction of the cloudy lens but, in virtually every case in this country, implantation of a clear, plastic **intraocular lens (IOL)** in its place to serve the same focusing function. We'll discuss the lens implant later in this section, but we note here that two tests are routinely carried out before surgery to craft the lens.

Both tests are conducted in order to estimate the power or prescription of the implant. The **A-scan** measures the length of your eye, using sound waves, while a **keratometer** measures the curvature of your cornea.

Q: In other words, people get the same *impaired* vision they had before they got cataracts?

A: More or less. Most people who undergo cataract surgery still need glasses or contact lenses to correct such conditions as myopia and presbyopia—the refractive errors discussed in Chapter 2—although the glasses will probably fine-tune their vision rather than make major corrections.

Surgical Approaches

Q: So how is a cataract removed?

A: There are three main types of cataract surgery: intracapsular, extracapsular and **phacoemulsification (PE)**, which is actually a variation of extracapsular and is the state-of-the-art procedure these days.

For decades the intracapsular method, in which the lens is removed in its entirety, was the standard form of cataract surgery. However, advances in microsurgery have made it obsolete, and it's now performed primarily in developing countries.

Q: Which method uses a laser?

A: Contrary to popular misconception, lasers aren't used to remove cataracts. But, as we discuss later, they are often used after the cataract is extracted, to remove an opacity that's the most common adverse effect of this surgery. More about that before the end of this chapter.

Q: What happens in extracapsular surgery?

A: First, you're anesthetized. In most cases you're given a mild sedative, usually intravenously, and then local anesthesia to numb the eye, block pain and prevent you from closing and moving your eye during surgery.

Next, your pupil is dilated as much as possible to expose more of the cataract. Then, using a scalpel under an operating microscope, the ophthalmologist makes a small incision into the eye to gain access to the lens. The cataract is removed in parts, with the back or posterior part of the capsule—the thin membrane that completely surrounds the lens—left behind to help support the implant.

The relatively small incision—less than half an inch—is big enough for the hard nucleus to be removed in one piece. The remaining cortex—the soft area between the outer capsule and inner nucleus—is aspirated, or sucked out. The surgeon closes the incision with stitches.

Q: How does PE differ from that?

A: In PE the nucleus is not removed in one piece. Instead it's broken up and liquefied, or emulsified, by the minute vibrations of a handheld ultrasound probe. Then it's aspirated through a needle. The advantage of this method is that it permits the surgeon to make an incision only big enough to accommodate the probe—about one-eighth of an inch.

As a result the incision may be closed with only a few very small stitches. Increasingly, in fact, PE has become a "no-stitch" procedure: The surgeon makes the incision in the sclera, tunnels under it into the cornea and ends the incision in a corneal flap. Pressure of fluid in the eye forces the flap to seal itself.

Q: What's so important about eliminating stitches?

A: It makes the healing process faster and reduces the risk of astigmatism. Astigmatism occurs because the stitches used in cataract surgery pull on the cornea slightly, causing the round cornea to become slightly oval.

Q: Given the benefits, why wouldn't everyone choose PE?

A: It's not everyone's choice to make. Cataracts that are very advanced and hard may be difficult to emulsify, so traditional extracapsular extraction may be the only option.

Ultimately the choice may not be that significant. "Six months or a year after surgery, there is generally little difference in the results between extracapsular cataract surgery and phacoemulsification," Shulman notes in *Cataracts*.

Q: Are there any recent innovations in cataract surgery?

A: As long as they have their patients under the knife, some surgeons are starting to combine cataract surgery with keratotomy, the procedure we described in Chapter 2, to correct astigmatisms.

Q: What happens after the cataract is removed? Does the plastic lens gets inserted?

A: That's right. At this point the individual has what's known as **aphakia**—an eye without a lens. As we noted in Chapter 1, the lens accounts for about 40 percent of the eye's refractive power. So, even without the cataract, vision will remain extremely blurry unless something is substituted for the natural lens.

Until 40 years ago, when contact lenses became available, aphakia was corrected with thick glasses that grossly magnified and distorted images. Now, however, virtually every cataract extraction is followed with the implantation of a plastic lens, usually in the space between the iris and the vitreous humor.

Q: Do you mean it's not attached in any discernible fashion?

A: It's held in place by two springlike fibers. To picture it, imagine a contact lens with a question mark extending from the top and bottom.

Q: Is there only one type of lens?

A: No, and the designs are being continually modified and improved. Most lenses are about one-quarter of an inch in diameter. As you may recall, extraction by phacoemulsification requires a one-eighth of an inch incision—an achievement that's lost if the incision must be widened to accommodate the lens. As a result surgeons have been developing implants that are oval or foldable—a silicone lens that can be squeezed into place—to preserve the advantage of small-incision surgery.

In addition intraocular lenses that are bifocal or trifocal—just like eyeglasses—to correct different types of refractive errors are now available. However, they're not yet widely used.

Q: How long does the entire procedure take?

A: Only about half an hour. Cataract surgery is almost always performed on an outpatient basis, with the entire visit typically taking no more than three hours.

Q: What's the recovery period like?

A: As far as their vision permits, people can generally return to normal activities the next day, although they shouldn't do anything strenuous for a couple of weeks. Some surgeons recommend that their patients wear a plastic or metal shield at bedtime to avoid rubbing the eye. Stitches, if any, rarely need to be removed.

Q: How soon does vision come back?

A: Usually vision is fully restored within a matter of weeks, but there's enormous variation, depending on a patient's response to the surgery. Postoperative vision may be excellent the next day or it may be even worse than before surgery, due to normal inflammation and clouding of the cornea and temporary bleeding. It may take as long as three to four months to fully improve.

Q: How successful is cataract surgery?

A: Extremely. It's generally reported that cataract surgery improves vision in 90 to 95 percent of all cases, although that doesn't mean that acuity is restored to 20/20. In fact, most people who undergo cataract surgery can expect to wear eyeglasses or contact lenses for the rest of their lives.

According to the Clinical Practice Guideline panel, "Corrected visual acuity in the 20/40 to 20/15 range is a reasonable expectation for the vast majority of patients," regardless of which procedure is used. "Generally patients can expect an increase in well-being and quality of life 90 percent of the time."

Q: Is the surgery safe?

A: There are risks, but the odds of something going very wrong are quite low.

About 1 percent of people who undergo cataract surgery develop a torn retina within half a year after the procedure. If caught early, this can be promptly repaired using the procedure described in Chapter 3.

There's also a very small risk of cystoid macular edema, the leakage of fluid from capillaries in the macula. Generally this can be treated with anti-inflammatory eyedrops.

In addition, an estimated 5,400 patients each year develop a bacterial eye infection known as **endophthalmitis** after surgery.

Q: How is the infection treated?

A: The traditional treatment has often been a combination of intravenous antibiotics and a vitrectomy—the surgical procedure, described in detail in the previous chapter, in which vitreous body and blood are removed and replaced with gas or other substances.

However, the NEI recently advised doctors that these infections can be treated adequately and cost effectively by injecting antibiotics into the vitreous material. The NEI also said that a vitrectomy benefits only those individuals whose vision is extremely low—about 25 percent of patients—and should not be performed on the overwhelming majority.

Q: Can a cataract come back?

A: No, because all or part of the lens has been removed. Many people may think a cataract is returning when the posterior capsule—the thin back membrane of the original cataract that is left in the eye to hold the implant in place—begins to cloud over, bringing back cataract symptoms such as blurred vision and glare.

This is the most common adverse result of cataract surgery, occurring about 25 percent of the time. Technically it isn't a complication, because it's a natural consequence of cataract surgery as it's performed today.

Complication or not, **posterior capsular opacification**, as it's called, can reduce vision within a couple of years to the point where it's as bad as if the original cataract had never been removed.

Q: Can it be treated?

A: That's where lasers come in. Most surgeons today use a YAG (yttrium aluminum garnet) laser to create a small opening in the center of the posterior capsule. The procedure, known as **YAG laser capsulotomy**, is performed with a topical anesthetic to the cornea, on an outpatient basis.

The procedure restores vision promptly in about two-thirds of patients, according to a review of medical literature by the Clinical Practice Guideline panel.

Q: Is a laser capsulotomy safe?

A: Overall, yes. Probably the greatest concern is the slightly increased risk of retinal detachment, the vision-threatening condition discussed in Chapter 3. An analysis of nearly 14,000 Medicare patient records by the Cataract Patient Outcomes Research Team indicates that patients who underwent YAG capsulotomy had four times the risk of a detached retina of those who didn't.

Because that was somewhat higher than had been expected,

it may lead doctors and patients to defer YAG laser surgery until vision is poor enough to warrant the risk.

In addition, there's a slight long-term risk that laser capsulotomy could lead to glaucoma by triggering a rise in **intraocular pressure**. For more information about glaucoma, see Chapter 5.

Q: Are there any other side effects of cataract surgery?

A: You may have eye pain or irritation, dry eye, redness, tearing or double vision, but usually these symptoms go away as inflammation subsides. Sometimes the cataract extraction itself causes a change in the pressure in the eye, a serious risk for anyone with glaucoma.

Initially, too, your eyes may be extremely sensitive to light. That's partly because you're so unused to seeing clearly and partly because the iris is inflamed and becomes irritable when it has to adjust to bright light.

This is a temporary reaction, though. In fact, most of the intraocular lenses being implanted today contain ultraviolet filters that reduce sensitivity. People with the older lenses may protect their eyes from ultraviolet rays with oversized, wraparound sunglasses.

Q: If I've got cataracts in both eyes, should I have them removed at the same time?

A: "In no case should surgery be done on both eyes in the same surgical procedure," is the unequivocal conclusion of the Clinical Practice Guideline panel. The reason is to avert catastrophe in the highly unlikely event that either the instruments or materials used in the procedure prove to be unsterile.

Q: Then how long should I wait between operations?

A: That depends on you, your surgeon and your insurance policy. A waiting period of six to eight weeks is common.

It's worth noting that at least one health insurer has tried to limit reimbursement to only one cataract removal, even for people with cataracts in both eyes. The effort was unsuccessful, but in this era of managed care, it may be tried again. However, the panel, noting the significant disabilities caused by one bad eye, strongly endorsed the potential benefit of surgery on the second eye.

5 GLAUCOMA

Q: What is glaucoma?

A: It's a disease of the optic nerve, that bundle of nerves that carries images from the retina to the brain. In most cases of glaucoma, the normal fluid pressure inside the eyes, known as the intraocular pressure (IOP), slowly rises, putting direct pressure on optic nerve fibers. Untreated, the disease may lead to vision loss, as the fibers die, or even to blindness.

Q: Why does IOP increase?

A: As we mentioned in Chapter 1, the space between the iris and cornea is filled with a clear solution, called the aqueous humor, that's produced by ciliary tissues around the lens.

Normally this fluid flows out of the inner part of the eye through the pupil and then is absorbed into the bloodstream through the **trabecular meshwork**—the system of tiny drainage canals all around the outer edge of the iris. The continual production, flow and drainage help bathe and nourish the lens, iris and cornea. (Don't confuse this fluid with tears, which cover the outer surface of the eye.)

With the most common type of glaucoma, **open-angle glaucoma**, the fluid drains too slowly out of the eye. With the far less common type, **closed-angle glaucoma**, the drainage canals may be blocked altogether.

Q: Open angle? Closed angle? What's that all about?

A: That refers to the angle where the iris meets the cornea. In open-angle glaucoma the angle is as wide and open as it should be, and the entrances to the drainage canals are clear. The problem is that the drainage canals are clogged inside, much as the pipe below the drain of a sink can clog. About 90 percent of people with glaucoma have this type.

With closed-angle glaucoma the angle between the iris and the cornea is not as wide and open as it should be. So when the pupil enlarges too much or too quickly, the outer edge of the iris impinges on the drainage canals. In plumbing terms the drainage canals are actually blocked or covered over, just as if a piece of plastic covered the drain of a sink.

Q: So open-angle glaucoma develops more gradually?

A: That's right. It's a chronic, or long-term, condition. It progresses very slowly as the eye's drainage canals become more and more clogged and pressure within the eye gradually increases.

Usually this buildup happens without any pain or discomfort. It may take years before there's any visual change, and when it occurs it's likely to be so slight—and limited to the periphery—that it may go unnoticed until there's a lot of irreversible optic nerve damage and the field of vision has significantly narrowed.

Q: What happens in closed-angle glaucoma?

A: That's an acute condition, in which things can take a sudden change for the worse. Symptoms and damage are usually very noticeable: blurred vision, severe headaches or eye pain, nausea and vomiting, rainbow halos around lights at night.

Q: Why do the drainage canals stop functioning properly?

A: Age seems to be the culprit in the case of open-angle glaucoma, as in so many other vision-threatening disorders. But no one knows why older people develop this condition.

"It is not clear whether older eyes are more susceptible to injury or whether they have simply had longer exposure to other risk factors such as high intraocular pressure," Harry A. Quigley, M.D., of the Wilmer Ophthalmological Institute at Johns Hopkins University School of Medicine, Baltimore, wrote in a review article in the *New England Journal of Medicine*.

As for closed-angle glaucoma, that's a rare structural problem. It can be triggered when the pupil is enlarged by certain medications, or by entry into a darkened room or movie theater, for instance.

Q: Is glaucoma likely to affect both eyes?

A: It usually occurs in both eyes, but the IOP often builds up first in one eye.

Q: Are there other types of glaucoma?

A: Yes, there are many. **Secondary glaucoma** can occur as the result of an eye injury, inflammation or tumor, in which the outflow of aqueous humor is impaired. This glaucoma may be acute or chronic.

Neovascular glaucoma can occur in people with retinal vascular disease, particularly diabetic retinopathy.

Congenital glaucoma occurs in infants. This very rare condition may be inherited and is the result of incorrect or incomplete development of the eye's drainage canals during prenatal development.

Q: And you can get glaucoma without high intraocular pressure?

A: Yes. While high IOP has come to be equated with glaucoma, there are numerous cases where people with high IOP never develop glaucoma. For example, women tend to have higher eye pressure than men but not a higher rate of glaucoma. And, on the other hand, many people with normal IOP have the sort of optic nerve damage associated with glaucoma.

In fact, in some surveys between 25 and 50 percent of people with glaucomatous damage to the optic nerve have normal IOP. Other sources indicate that this condition, known as **normal-tension glaucoma**, is rare.

Q: If IOP isn't always the culprit, what else causes glaucoma?

A: Some researchers suspect that certain conditions may make some people particularly susceptible to glaucoma. In one small study, Swiss researchers found that glaucoma patients with visual damage had lower systolic blood pressure—that is, a lower value for the upper number—

than a control group.

In the March 1996 *Archives of Ophthalmology*, researchers at the Massachusetts Eye and Ear Infirmary, Boston, and Harvard Medical School suggested that excessive levels of glutamate—an amino acid known to be toxic, in high concentrations, to optic nerve cells—may also be responsible for destroying sight. They speculated that the disease begins with increased fluid in the eye. The higher pressure crushes a few of the nerve cells in the retina, releasing toxic levels of glutamate.

Q: Is glaucoma common?

A: Very. According to the National Eye Institute (NEI), about 2 million people in the United States have glaucoma and 80,000 are blind from open-angle glaucoma. However, given the insidious nature of the disease, it's thought that far more people may have glaucoma without knowing it.

After macular degeneration and cataracts, glaucoma is the third leading cause of blindness in the United States. It's also the second leading cause of irreversible blindness, after macular degeneration.

Q: Who gets glaucoma?

A: Glaucoma can affect anyone, but it's most common in people over age 60. It is also common in African Americans older than 40. Five times more prevalent among African Americans than whites, glaucoma is the leading cause of blindness among African Americans. Why they should be at higher risk is unclear, although they do have a higher prevalence of elevated blood pressure and IOP.

A related statistic is that glaucoma is 15 times more likely to cause blindness in African Americans between ages 45 and 64 than in whites of the same age group. And blindness due to open-angle glaucoma is about six times more common among

African Americans than among white Americans. According to
the NEI, that statistic reflects not only the fact that African
Americans are less likely to receive timely treatment but also
that their disease is more severe.

Q: Any other risk factors?

A: Apart from age and race, the main risk factors include
a family history of glaucoma, although the pattern of
inheritance is unclear; past injuries to the eyes; diabetes; and
regular use of corticosteroids (especially as eyedrops), which
raise IOP.

In addition, in some studies high blood pressure and
smoking were found to be risk factors for glaucoma, or at least
for high IOP. Extreme nearsightedness or farsightedness also
plays a minor role.

And, as a medical curiosity, we'll add one small group for
whom glaucoma may be an occupational hazard: brass musicians. In a 1995 study, Theodore Krupin, M.D., an ophthalmologist at Northwestern University Medical School, Chicago,
found that eye pressure increases when musicians strain to
force air through their horns.

Brief strains are not harmful, but the problem is more
serious with professional musicians, who may practice several
hours a day. Krupin found that the pressure rise was most
pronounced in trumpeters and French horn players.

Q: Does having cataracts put me at increased risk for glaucoma?

A: No. They often occur together simply because they
both develop as people age. However, cataract surgery
can cause a change in the IOP; it may go up or down, and the
change may be permanent or temporary. Doctors closely
monitor their glaucoma patients after cataract surgery for
"pressure spikes," or sharp increases in IOP.

EXAMINATION

Q: How is glaucoma detected?

A: The primary test for glaucoma is **tonometry**, which measures the IOP.

This may be done with an air tonometer, which directs a puff of air against the eye and measures the time it takes to flatten the cornea. However, this has been largely superseded by newer types of tonometers. After numbing the eye with anesthetic drops, the practitioner presses the instrument lightly against the cornea. The pressure causes a slight indentation, and the tonometer registers the eye's resistance.

Q: What is considered a high IOP?

A: Because, as we indicated earlier, not all high IOPs are linked to glaucoma and not all glaucomas are linked to high IOPs, it's a somewhat ambiguous measure. However, "normal" pressures usually range from 12 to 22 mm Hg, or millimeters of mercury, which is a scale for recording eye pressure.

As we said, women typically have slightly higher pressures than men, and Asians have lower pressures than whites or African Americans.

Q: Since pressure isn't always meaningful, are there other tests?

A: The other standard diagnostic test is ophthalmoscopy, a test that allows the practitioner to see whether the optic nerve has been damaged. A damaged nerve will have a "cupped" disc shape—a concavity created by the higher pressure—and its tissue is pale, in contrast to the normal pink of healthy tissue.

The practitioner may also use a slit-lamp microscope, described in Chapter 1, which lets him inspect the drainage system and optic nerve for signs of damage.

If pressures are high or the optic nerve looks unusual, most doctors do one or two special glaucoma tests: **perimetry** and **gonioscopy**.

Q: What happens in perimetry?

A: Perimetry is a test that produces a map of the complete field of vision. It's useful because it detects very small changes in peripheral vision, where glaucoma makes its first inroads.

State-of-the art testing is done through automated visual field analysis: A computer flashes points of light around a bowl-shaped area while the individual touches a switch as soon as he thinks he sees the light, however dim. The test is a highly sensitive early detector.

Q: And what does gonioscopy involve?

A: After numbing your cornea, the practitioner places on your eye a handheld contact lens. This allows him to look sideways into your eye to check whether the angle where the iris meets the cornea is open (open-angle glaucoma) or closed (closed-angle glaucoma).

Q: How often should I be examined?

A: That depends on your age, your race and other risk factors, and what the tests—if you've had them already—have shown.

According to the American Academy of Ophthalmology, if you're over 40, you should be examined routinely for glaucoma every three to five years. You should be examined every year or two if you're African American, have a blood relative with glaucoma, have had a serious eye injury in the past or are taking steroids.

Q: And how often should I be examined if I already have glaucoma?

A: If you've been diagnosed with glaucoma, your IOP will initially be checked every week or so until it's under control. Even when it's at a safe level, you may need to see your doctor several times a year for checkups.

One drawback to such tests is that eye pressures vary at different times of the day. Aqueous flow is highest in the early waking hours and lowest during the night. Improved self-tonometry devices to be used at home are being developed that should help people monitor their intraocular pressures.

In addition, you need a visual field test once or twice a year, to ensure that your field of vision isn't changing.

TREATMENT

Q: When is glaucoma treated?

A: Glaucoma is diagnosed and treatment is started if the pressure in both eyes is over 30 mm Hg and the optic nerve is cupped, or if the visual field map shows some abnormal patterns that are typical of glaucoma damage.

But often the signs are more ambiguous, and treatment is a tough judgment call. For example, an individual's IOP may be between 22 and 30 mm Hg, but the optic nerve and visual field show no signs of damage. As we indicated, some people have high IOP for years and their sight is never affected. In such borderline cases, practitioners may look for clues, including slight changes in the optic nerve or a history of glaucoma in the patient's family.

Sometimes eye care practitioners withhold treatment from people with mildly or moderately elevated IOP until there's evidence of glaucomatous damage. They do this because only a small proportion of patients actually develop damage and, as we discuss in this section, the cost and adverse side effects of treatment are considerable.

On the other hand, many clinicians immediately prescribe medication in a desire to prevent any damage to the optic nerve.

Q: How is glaucoma treated?

A: Glaucoma has historically been linked to high IOP, and IOP remains a major cause of the condition. So the main objective of treatment is to lower IOP, either by decreasing the amount of aqueous humor that's produced or by increasing its outflow.

For open-angle glaucoma, that's typically done with medication—usually eyedrops, sometimes eyedrops and pills together. However, recent research has established that laser therapy may be more effective. Another option is microsurgery.

Next we describe the several categories of medication you can expect to receive. However, keep in mind that because treatment for glaucoma is lifelong, it's likely that a certain type or dosage may lose its effectiveness from time to time and a different drug will be prescribed. Furthermore, new medications to treat glaucoma are continually being developed.

Q: Okay. What medications are most commonly prescribed?

A: The most commonly prescribed drugs for glaucoma are beta blockers, which decrease IOP by slowing the production of aqueous humor. Beta blockers include timolol (Timoptic, made by Merck) and betaxolol (Betoptic, by Alcon).

The second category is the epinephrine-related drugs, which increase the outflow of aqueous humor. These include epinephrine (Epifrin, by Allergan) and dipivefrin (Propine, also by Allergan).

Both types of drugs, all in eyedrop form, are preferred because they are effective and may be taken only twice daily, as opposed to other drugs that must be taken four times daily.

Q: What other types of medications are available?

A: The third major category of medication is **miotics**, which decrease pressure by tightening the muscles that close the pupil, thus stretching the trabecular meshwork.

Miotics include pilocarpine (Ocusert, made by Alza) and pilocarpine hydrochloride (Pilopine HS, made by Alcon). Like the first two types, they're delivered in eyedrop form. Partly because they must be taken four times a day, they're not prescribed as often as the other two groups.

The fourth category is **carbonic anhydrase inhibitors**, which suppress production of aqueous humor. They include acetazolamide (Diamox, made by Lederle) and methazolamide (Neptazane, also from Lederle), both in pill form, and dorzolamide hydrochloride (Trusopt, made by Merck), an eyedrop.

Finally, at the end of 1995 an advisory panel recommended that the Food and Drug Administration approve a new type of drug to battle glaucoma. The drug, Latanoprost, made by Pharmacia Upjohn, is the first of a new class of drugs based on a natural chemical, prostaglandin, that helps the eye drain off its fluid.

Q: Do these medications have side effects?

A: Unfortunately glaucoma medications often cause both physical and emotional changes that are unpleasant or even serious.

The first group, beta blockers, can cause breathing problems for people with asthma or emphysema. They may contribute to irregular heart rhythm and, in elderly people, to congestive heart failure. More common effects—occurring in perhaps 25 percent of people who take them—include mental and physical lethargy, depression, memory loss and a decrease in libido, or sex drive.

The epinephrine-related drugs can cause rapid or irregular heartbeat and high blood pressure, as well as headache, tremor and restlessness. Because they make the pupils larger, people who also have cataracts may notice an increase in glare.

Miotics, because they constrict the pupils, can lead to blurred vision and poor night vision. Other side effects include nearsightedness, watering eyes, brow- and eyeaches, and allergic reactions.

Q: What about the pills?

A: The carbonic anhydrase inhibitors have their own set of side effects: lethargy, appetite suppression and itchy or burning skin. What's more disturbing is that they've also been associated with kidney stones and aplastic anemia, a blood cell disorder.

Furthermore, this class of medications may cause intolerable side effects in up to half of patients, roughly double the rate of the other categories of medication for glaucoma. So they're generally used only when glaucoma isn't controlled by the eyedrops.

Q: Is the new drug, based on prostaglandin, any better?

A: Yes and no. In studies it worked better than standard therapy and produced significantly fewer side effects. However, it did have one startling side effect: In 16 percent of patients who used the drug for a year, it turned blue or green eyes to brown.

The change is apparently irreversible, but it's unknown whether it's dangerous. No other drug or agent has ever been found to produce this result.

Q: What if none of the medications helps?

A: When medications don't help or, as is often the case, people fail to take them as often as they should, doctors have traditionally turned to laser surgery as a "next-best" therapy for open-angle glaucoma. In fact, recent research indicates that early laser treatment may be the best approach for this type of glaucoma.

Q: What happens in laser therapy?

A: In a procedure known as a **trabeculoplasty**, an ophthalmologist uses an argon laser to burn 100 tiny holes in the trabecular meshwork. These burns stretch the existing holes in the meshwork, allowing the aqueous humor to drain faster from the eye.

Q: Is it effective?

A: According to a seven-year study sponsored by the NEI and published in the *American Journal of Ophthalmology* in 1995, initial treatment with laser is at least as effective as initial treatment with medication. And because it's relatively noninvasive, it's also quite safe.

The researchers found that two years after treatment, 56 percent of the eyes that had received laser therapy first required medication later to control pressure, while 70 percent of eyes that were started on medication required new or added medication in the same period.

Moreover, the laser-treated eyes that eventually required drug therapy needed less medication than did the eyes treated initially with drugs alone.

Q: But ultimately more treatment is required?

A: Sooner or later the drains close up again and, since they can be treated only once by laser, will require medication or traditional microsurgery.

Q: What happens in microsurgery?

A: First, to prevent any future problems with acute glaucoma, a tiny piece of the iris is removed in a preventive **iridectomy**. Then, in a procedure called a **trabeculectomy**, or **sclerostomy**, the surgeon makes a tiny opening in the sclera, the white part of the eye. This new opening allows the aqueous humor to bypass the clogged drainage canals.

As the fluid flows out of this new, artificial drainage canal, the tissue over the opening rises to form a little blister or bubble, called a **bleb**. The bleb, which will be a color slightly different from the white sclera, indicates that the canal is draining properly.

Q: Is a trabeculectomy effective?

A: Yes, usually. In a study cited in the *New England Journal of Medicine*, five years after the operation, 75 percent of treated eyes still have good IOP and no complications. However, the risk of permanent loss of vision due to surgery may be 5 percent, and about 1 percent of people develop bacterial infections. There's also a risk of cataracts.

Furthermore, in some cases—typically younger people—the new drainage canal begins to close because the body is trying to heal the "wound," and the pressure rises again. If necessary, a trabeculectomy can be done several times in the same eye.

Q: Is the procedure being improved?

A: Yes. One study has demonstrated that the drug 5-fluorouracil (better-known to ophthalmologists as 5-FU), which prevents scar tissue from forming, can improve the outcome of microsurgery and reduce the need for further surgery or daily medications.

It's particularly helpful with people for whom a trabeculectomy might otherwise fail because they've already had either cataract surgery or an unsuccessful trabeculectomy.

Q: Is there a different treatment for acute closed-angle and congenital glaucomas?

A: The treatment of choice is a procedure called a laser **iridotomy**. After the glaucoma has been temporarily controlled with medication, the surgeon creates a tiny opening in the iris so the aqueous fluid can drain better. This is generally the only way that the blocked or incorrectly formed drainage canals can be opened up.

Q: Is the procedure effective?

A: Yes, in the early stages of acute closed-angle glaucoma. Congenital glaucoma is harder to treat.

Q: With all this surgery, what does the eye look like?

A: It generally looks completely normal, whether the procedure has been done by laser or traditional microsurgery. The opening in the iris made in an iridotomy is barely visible, while the new drainage canal created in a trabeculectomy is usually hidden under the upper eyelid. You can see it if you gently pull your eyelid up near the eyebrow and tilt your head back a little while looking in a mirror.

Q: If those procedures don't work, are there any others?

A: Yes. One alternative involves improving the outflow of aqueous humor through a shunt, or implanted artificial drainage system made out of plastic tubing. The other involves decreasing the production of aqueous humor by selectively destroying the ciliary body, by either freezing or laser.

However, both these procedures are still under study and are risky; the latter option may lead to a decrease in vision in 25 percent of patients, according to Quigley's *New England Journal of Medicine* article. So they're normally reserved for severe, uncontrolled glaucoma.

Q: All those treatments deal with reducing IOP. What if that isn't the cause?

A: It's still the target. According to the NEI, recent studies report that progressive glaucoma damage in most patients can be inhibited by reducing IOP to a level lower than previously thought to be needed.

Q: Can I do anything myself to beat glaucoma?

A: There are no hard data that would mandate changes in diet or behavior, but there are indications that you can in fact help control your glaucoma with certain behaviors (in addition to taking your medicine).

Regular aerobic exercise has been shown to lower IOP in some cases. Other studies have found that high blood pressure and smoking are risk factors. Although there are no controlled data to support it, Quigley wrote in the *New England Journal of Medicine*, "medical treatment of vascular disease and the cessation of smoking may be presumed to be reasonable interventions."

And researchers are investigating the possibility that open-angle glaucoma, like so many eye and other disorders, may be controlled or prevented by consuming antioxidant nutrients found in dark green leafy and yellow or red vegetables, such as broccoli, spinach and carrots.

Q: Isn't marijuana supposed to help control glaucoma?

A: There's strong anecdotal evidence that smoking marijuana lowers IOP, but no reliable research to date—and, so far, no success in getting it legalized for that use.

Q: So there's nothing more I can do to prevent glaucoma?

A: New drugs are coming onto the market at an unprecedented rate, and treatments like laser surgery are undergoing rapid improvement. According to Anne Sumers, M.D., a general ophthalmologist in Ridgewood, New Jersey, and a spokesperson for the American Academy of Ophthalmology, "If you're got to have glaucoma, you couldn't have chosen a better point in time."

In the meanwhile get your eyes checked regularly.

6 OTHER QUESTIONS ABOUT THE EYE

Q: Are there any other conditions that threaten vision?

A: Yes. In this chapter we'll discuss a number of other diseases and disorders, some of which we have mentioned previously but haven't addressed at length. We'll also discuss them and their treatments, as well as nonmedical devices for improving low vision.

Amid all this talk of disease, however, let's not lose sight of one of the most significant sources of vision problems, particularly in the young: accidents. Over 1 million people, more than half of whom are under the age of 25, suffer eye injuries each year in the United States. And, according to the American Academy of Ophthalmology (AAO), 90 percent of these eye injuries could have been prevented.

Almost half of these accidents occurred at home. Causes? Everything from the misuse of household cleaning products and garden tools to playing with fireworks and projectile toys.

For a first-aid chart and brochures on how to prevent eye injuries, contact the AAO. (See the Informational and Mutual-Aid Groups section of this book.)

OTHER VISION-THREATENING CONDITIONS

Q: What other conditions can jeopardize vision?

A: According to the National Eye Institute (NEI), at least 8,000 Americans each year develop a condition called **nonarteritic ischemic optic neuropathy**. It's the most common cause of sudden vision loss in people 60 and older, but many under the age of 60 also develop the condition.

The neuropathy results from a painless swelling of the optic nerve, which connects the eye and the brain. No one knows what causes the swelling, but it comes on so suddenly that those affected by it often awake blinded in one eye. In 40 percent of those affected, both eyes may ultimately be affected.

Q: How is it treated?

A: Until recently, the treatment of choice was a surgical procedure called optic nerve decompression, in which an ophthalmologist cuts through the eye muscles to reach behind the eye and make two or more slits in the sheath surrounding the optic nerve. This allows the escape of cerebrospinal fluid. In the past at least 1,000 such operations have been performed each year.

However, a study sponsored by the NEI recently reported that the procedure was ineffective and possibly harmful. The study found that individuals who had no treatment at all recovered their vision after a period of six months at a rate considerably higher than those who had the surgery. Furthermore, those who had surgery had a greater loss of visual acuity than those who had no treatment.

As a result, in 1995 federal health officials warned eye surgeons against the procedure.

Q: Are there other diseases that affect the optic nerve?

A: Arteriosclerosis, or hardening of the arteries, can result in insufficient blood flow to the optic nerve, causing sudden loss of vision.

Q: Apart from the retina, where do tumors occur in the eye?

A: Tumors can be found in the eyelids, in surrounding tissues and related structures, as well as in the retina. Tumors affecting the eyes include:

- Eyelid tumors. These are quite common and look like irregularities or bumps. Although usually benign, they can occasionally be malignant. The only way to determine for sure is to examine the tissue under a microscope. If the tumor is small, your ophthalmologist may recommend removing it completely.

- Conjunctival tumors. These usually appear as lumpy or slightly raised areas against the white background. Malignant tumors are extremely rare but, if they're suspected, must be either removed surgically or radiated promptly.

- Orbital tumors. Tumors may arise in the socket behind the eye, displacing the eyeball and causing decreased or double vision. Diagnosis usually requires extensive evaluation and often includes x-rays and blood tests. Treatment may include radiation therapy or surgical removal of the tumor.

Q: What else can cause vision loss?

A: In Chapter 2 we described the major infections that can affect the cornea and even lead to blindness.

A number of other diseases and disorders, although less common, can also damage the cornea.

In fact, disease and injury to the cornea are the leading cause of visits to physicians for eye care in the United States, according to the NEI, and corneal diseases are an ophthalmological subspecialty.

Q: Besides infection, what conditions can damage the cornea?

A: One of the more common is **keratoconus,** a non-inflammatory, progressive thinning of the cornea that leads to a distortion of its curvature, so that the cornea assumes a conical shape. The problem first shows up in young adults; vision becomes mildly blurred or distorted, and can't be corrected by eyeglasses.

Keratoconus has been associated with wearing contact lenses for long periods. It also occurs in people with Down syndrome.

Another condition is corneal dystrophy, in which—due to genetic inheritance—alterations occur in the cornea. The most common is **Fuchs' dystrophy,** a disorder of the corneal endothelium, the innermost layer of the cornea. In this condition, which occurs mostly in the elderly, the cornea swells and vision becomes blurred.

Q: Doesn't the cornea get injured, too?

A: Yes, through surgery—typically cataract extractions, as we mentioned in Chapter 4—and other trauma, including accidents. Corneas also get burned from intense light sources—arc welding equipment, tanning lights or the sun during a solar eclipse. Gazing at them can cause a painful corneal condition called **photokeratitis,** and even a permanent loss of central vision.

Q: What happens if the cornea doesn't heal?

A: One recourse—used on approximately 120,000 eyes annually in the United States, according to the NEI—is a corneal transplant. This involves replacing the central section of the cornea—generally a disc eight millimeters in diameter—with a donated section of the same size and shape.

The transplant is sewn into place with microsurgical instruments. The actual surgery takes about one hour.

Q: Is corneal transplant successful?

A: Yes. In the words of the NEI's corneal diseases panel, transplantation "has restored sight to many who a generation ago would have been blinded permanently by corneal injury or infection, inherited corneal disease or corneal degeneration."

The main risk of failure is rejection of the new cornea, and that's relatively rare. The key to averting rejection, the Collaborative Corneal Transplantation Studies recently concluded, is donor/recipient blood matching and postoperative high-dose topical steroids.

Q: Where do the donated corneas come from?

A: From eye banks, which keep the eyes of people who have agreed to donate their eyes upon death. Only human donor material is used. Since the cornea is clear, the color of the donor's eye doesn't matter—nor, interestingly enough, does the visual acuity.

Q: Can the entire eye be transplanted?

A: Medical science hasn't yet developed a way to transplant a whole eye. The reason is that the optic nerve cannot be reconnected once it's severed. Because of this, the eye is never removed from its socket during surgery.

LOW VISION DEVICES

Q: Apart from conventional glasses, are there any optical aids for people with low vision?

A: There are many such devices, and often two or more will be prescribed to enable an individual to perform different tasks. Here's a list of those most often recommended:

- Magnifying spectacles. These are high-powered magnifying lenses that can be worn for reading, writing and other close work.

- Handheld magnifiers. These are simple magnifying glasses, in a variety of shapes and powers, that can be used for such tasks as reading price tags. There are also stand magnifiers for reading for longer periods of time. Both can be equipped with lights.

- Telescopes. Used for distant and intermediate seeing. Those mounted in eyeglass frames may be used for watching sports events or movies. Handheld telescopes, which generally have a wider range of power and a larger field of view, may be used for such tasks as spotting bus numbers. The telemicroscope—a telescope with a reading, or near-vision, lens—is used for intermediate seeing tasks such as using a computer or reading music.

- Field expanders. Used to increase the field of view, these devices consist of a small mirror, a partial prism or a telescope mounted backward. Depending on the visual field loss involved, they can be attached to an eyeglass frame or lens on one side or at the top or bottom.

- Closed-circuit TV (CCTV). This technology enlarges material on a video screen, producing an electronic image that allows the user to adjust image brightness, size, contrast and background illumination. CCTVs are expensive, however, running into the thousands of dollars, and are less portable than other magnifiers.

Q: **Is there anything specifically for night vision problems?**

A: Yes, night vision aids (NVAs), which take the available light in the environment and amplify it. NVAs have recently taken great strides technologically, thanks partly to the demands of the military in the Persian Gulf War.

Because they restrict the field of vision, NVAs can be a problem for someone with retinitis pigmentosa whose peripheral vision is already limited. But they can be a useful way for people to scan their surroundings and get their bearings.

For a list of distributors of night vision technology, write to the Foundation for Fighting Blindness. (See the Informational and Mutual-Aid Groups section of this book.)

Q: **Are there other aids or services?**

A: There's a wide variety of nonoptical materials and services, from large-type books and talking books to independent home-living instruction and mobility training. Many government and private agencies provide social services for people with low vision.

For more information, contact the agencies listed in the Informational and Mutual-Aid Groups section of this book, as well as your local office of the state commission for the blind and visually impaired.

Q: **Is there any way I can get free eye care?**

A: If you're at least 65, a U.S. citizen or legal resident and financially disadvantaged, you probably qualify for the National Eye Care Project. Sponsored by the Foundation of the American Academy of Ophthalmology and state ophthalmological societies, it provides free medical eye care: a comprehensive eye examination and treatment for whatever condition or disease is diagnosed.

For more information, contact the National Eye Care Project Helpline. (See the Informational and Mutual-Aid Groups section of this book.)

While eyeglasses and prescription drugs are not covered by the AAO's project, free eyeglasses are often available through Lions Clubs International. To find out how to obtain a pair, contact your local chapter.

Whether it's free eye care or other services or products, there are many ways you can help yourself see better. Be sure to do everything you can to protect and preserve your eyesight—it's your most precious sense.

INFORMATIONAL
AND
MUTUAL-AID GROUPS

American Academy of Ophthalmology
P.O. Box 7424
San Francisco, CA 94120-7424
415-561-8500

American Diabetes Association
1660 Duke St.
Alexandria, VA 22314
800-232-3472

American Foundation for the Blind
11 Penn Plaza, Suite 300
New York, NY 10001
800-232-5463

American Optometric Association
243 N. Lindbergh Blvd.
St. Louis, MO 63141-7881
314-991-4100

Association for Macular Diseases
210 E. 64th St.
New York, NY 10021
212-605-3719

Foundation for Fighting Blindness
National Retinitis Pigmentosa Foundation
800-683-5555
800-683-5551
Retina bank 24-hour hotline: 800-638-1818

Glaucoma Research Foundation
490 Post St., Suite 830
San Francisco, CA 94102
800-826-6693

Lighthouse National Center for Vision and Aging
111 E. 59th St.
New York, NY 10022
800-334-5497

National Association for Visually Handicapped
22 W. 21st St.
New York, NY 10010
212-889-3141

National Eye Care Project Helpline
800-222-EYES

National Eye Health Education Program
National Eye Institute
National Institutes of Health
Box 20/20
Bethesda, MD 20892

**National Library Service for the Blind and
Physically Handicapped**
Library of Congress
Washington, DC 20542
800-424-8567

National Sjögren's Syndrome Association
P.O. Box 42207
Phoenix, AZ 85080
800-395-NSSA

Prevent Blindness America
500 E. Remington Rd.
Schaumburg, IL 60173
800-331-2020

Sjögren's Syndrome Foundation
300 N. Broadway
Jericho, NY 11753
516-933-6365
800-4SJOGREN

EYE TREATMENT CENTERS

*The Top 17 Hospitals in the Field of Ophthalmology**

1. **Johns Hopkins Hospital (Wilmer Eye Institute)**
   600 N.Wolfe St.
   Baltimore, MD 21287
   410-955-5000

2. **University of Miami (Bascom Palmer Eye Institute)**
   900 NW 17th St.
   Miami, FL 33136-1199
   305-326-6000

3. **Wills Eye Hospital**
   900 Walnut St.
   Philadelphia, PA 19107
   215-928-3000

4. **Massachusetts Eye and Ear Infirmary**
   243 Charles St.
   Boston, MA 02114
   617-523-7900

5. **University of California at Los Angeles Medical Center (Jules Stein Eye Institute)**
   10833 Le Conte Ave.
   Los Angeles, CA 90095
   310-825-9111

6. **University of Iowa Hospitals and Clinics**
   200 Howkins Dr.
   Iowa City, IA 52242
   319-356-1616

7. **Barnes Hospital**
   1 Barnes Hospital Plaza
   St. Louis, MO 63110
   314-362-5000

8. **University of California
   San Francisco Medical Center**
   505 Parnassus Ave.
   San Francisco, CA 94143-0001
   415-476-1000

9. **Mayo Clinic**
   200 SW First St.
   Rochester, MN 55905
   507-284-2511

10. **Duke University Medical Center**
    Erwin Road
    Durham, NC 27710
    919-684-8111

11. **Manhattan Eye, Ear and Throat Hospital**
    210 E. 64th St.
    New York, NY 10021-7498
    212-838-9200

12. **Doheny Eye Institute**
    1450 San Pablo St.
    Los Angeles, CA 90033
    213-342-6600

13. **New York Eye and Ear Infirmary**
    310 E. 14th St.
    New York, NY 10002-4200
    212-598-1313

14. **University of Michigan Medical Center**
    1500 E. Medical Center Dr.
    Ann Arbor, MI 48109
    313-936-4000

15. Baylor University Medical Center
3500 Gaston Ave.
Dallas, TX 75246-2088
214-820-0111

16. Emory University Hospital
1364 Clifton Rd., NE
Atlanta, GA 30322-0001
404-712-7021

17. University of Illinois Hospital and Clinics
1740 W. Taylor St.
Chicago, IL 60612-4389
312-996-3900

*Based on annual surveys of a geographic cross-section of 150 board-certified specialists.

Source: U.S. News & World Report: America's Best Hospitals (New York: John Wiley & Sons, 1996).

GLOSSARY

Accommodative esotropia: A common form of strabismus that occurs in farsighted children after the age of two.

Age-related macular degeneration (AMD): A disorder of the macula that affects central vision. It is part of the normal aging process and the leading cause of new cases of blindness in people age 65 and older. See also **Dry AMD** and **Neovascular AMD**.

Aldose reductase: An enzyme that converts glucose into a sugar alcohol and that may help trigger diabetic complications.

Amblyopia: The reduction of central vision in one eye; also known as *lazy eye*.

Amsler grid: A sheet of graph paper, with a dot at the center, used to test for macular degeneration.

Aphakia: The condition, characteristic of cataract surgery decades ago, in which the eye is without its lens.

Aqueous humor: The watery fluid that fills the space between the cornea and the lens, and provides some of the nutrition for the surrounding parts.

A-scan: A test, prior to cataract surgery, that uses sound waves to measure the length of the eye.

Astigmatism: Distorted vision due to variations in refractive power of different parts of the cornea.

Biomicroscope: See **Slit lamp**.

Bleb: The small blister or bubble that forms over the artificial drainage canal created in a trabeculectomy, to control glaucoma.

Blepharitis: An inflammation of the eyelids caused by bacteria in the skin at the base of the eyelashes.

Bruch's membrane: A thin film of tissue underneath the retinal pigment epithelium.

Capsule: The thin membrane that completely surrounds the lens of the eye.

Carbonic anhydrase inhibitors: A class of drugs sometimes prescribed for glaucoma; they work by suppressing production of aqueous humor.

Carotenoids: A class of yellow and red pigments, found in leafy green vegetables, that are believed to help prevent certain degenerative retinal diseases.

Cataract: A clouding of the lens of the eye or of its surrounding transparent membrane; the clouding obstructs the passage of light.

Choroid: The layer of blood vessels that underlies the retina.

Choroidal melanoma: A tumor, arising from pigmented cells of the choroid, that is the most common cancer of the eye.

Ciliary muscles: The thin band of muscles, lining the wall of the eye, that help the lens focus.

Closed-angle glaucoma: The less-common type of glaucoma, in which the canals that drain fluid from the eyes are completely blocked.

CMV (cytomegalovirus) retinitis: A viral, vision-threatening retinal infection, often found in people with acquired immune deficiency syndrome (AIDS).

Cones: Cells, concentrated in the macula, that are responsible for central and color vision.

Congenital glaucoma: A rare condition, occurring in infants, characterized by the incorrect or incomplete development of the eye's drainage canals.

Conjunctiva: The thin, transparent tissue covering the white of the eye and the lining of the eyelids.

Conjunctivitis: Inflammation of the conjunctiva—widely known as pinkeye—resulting from allergies, irritants and infections.

Contrast sensitivity: The ability to discern an object from its background.

Convergence insufficiency: Very small deviation in alignment of the eyes, typically for close work.

Cornea: The clear covering over the front of the eye that bends, or refracts, light rays to help the eye focus.

Cortex: Within the lens capsule, the large fibers running from top to bottom around the nucleus.

Cortical cataract: A type of cataract in which the outer shell of the lens becomes progressively more opaque.

Cryotherapy: A surgical approach, involving the application of a freezing probe, that is sometimes used to repair retinal tears.

Dacryocystorhinostomy: A surgical procedure to bypass a blocked tear duct and create a new outlet for tears.

Dacryostenosis: Blocked tear duct, often found in infants.

Detached retina: A separation within the retina between the photoreceptors and the retinal pigment epithelium.

Diabetic retinopathy: A sight-threatening condition, common in people with diabetes, in which the blood vessels in the retina are diseased.

Diplopia: Double vision.

Drusen: Deposits, containing complex lipids and calcium, that are linked to the development of macular degeneration.

Dry AMD: A type of age-related macular degeneration, or AMD, that is characterized by the slow breakdown and death of the layer of light-sensing, or photoreceptor, cells in the macula. See also **Age-related macular degeneration (AMD).**

Dry eye: A condition in which the eye does not produce enough tears to be comfortable.

Ectropion: A condition in which, as skin stretches with age, the lower eyelid droops downward and turns out.

Electroretinogram (ERG): A test for retinitis pigmentosa that measures the electrical current produced by the photoreceptors.

Emmetropization: The natural process by which the length of the eye adjusts to its focal power, so distant images are seen clearly.

Endophthalmitis: A bacterial eye infection that is sometimes a complication of cataract surgery.

Endothelium: The innermost layer of the cornea.

Entropion: A condition in which the eyelid turns inward, bringing the eyelashes and skin to rub against the eye.

Esotropia: The type of strabismus in which the eye turns inward.

Exotropia: The type of strabismus in which the eye turns outward.

Floater: A tiny clump of gel or cells inside the vitreous; it looks like a small speck in one's field of vision.

Fluorescein: Nontoxic dye used in certain eye examinations.

Fovea: The center of the macula.

Fuchs' dystrophy: A disorder of the corneal endothelium in which the cornea swells up and vision becomes blurred.

Galactosemia: A rare disease, in newborns, of extreme lactose intolerance, often leading to the development of cataracts.

Glaucoma: A condition characterized by optic nerve damage and loss of vision, often caused by high intraocular pressure.

Gonioscopy: A glaucoma test that examines the angle where the iris meets the cornea.

Herpetic keratitis: An infection of the cornea caused by herpes simplex virus type I.

Hyperopia: The ability to see far objects more clearly and readily than close objects; also known as farsightedness.

Intraocular lens (IOL): A clear, plastic lens that is inserted during cataract surgery to serve the same focusing function as the extracted lens.

Intraocular pressure (IOP): The fluid pressure inside the eye. People with glaucoma often have an elevated IOP.

Iridectomy: A procedure, prior to a trabeculectomy, in which a tiny piece of the iris is removed, to prevent any future problems with acute glaucoma.

Iridotomy: A laser procedure in which the surgeon makes a tiny opening in the iris, to control acute closed-angle glaucoma.

Iris: The color part of the eye. It opens and closes to control the amount of light that enters the eye.

Keratoconus: A noninflammatory, progressive thinning of the cornea that leads to a distortion of its curvature and ultimately to vision loss.

Keratometer: An instrument that measures the curvature of the cornea.

Lacrimal gland: The gland, located in the upper eyelid, that secretes tears onto the surface of the eye.

Lacrimal sac: The cavity, located under the skin on the side of the nose, through which tears drain.

Legal blindness: The condition defined by best corrected visual acuity of 20/200 or worse in the better eye, or peripheral vision narrowed to 20 degrees or less in the better eye.

Lens: The clear, flexible structure located directly behind the eye's pupil.

Levator: The muscle that lifts the eyelid.

Low vision: Visual acuity generally defined as between 20/60 and 20/200 in the better eye, with corrective lenses.

Macula: Central area of the retina responsible for sharp, fine vision.

Macular degeneration: Damage or breakdown of the macula.

Macular edema: Swelling of the macula.

Microaneurysms: Small, pathological bulges on the blood vessels in the eye.

Miotics: A class of drugs, used for glaucoma, that decreases pressure by stretching the trabecular meshwork.

Myopia: The inability to see clearly at a distance; also known as nearsightedness.

Neovascular AMD: A condition in which abnormal new blood vessels grow under the retina, leaking fluid and damaging the macula; also known as wet AMD. See also **Age-related macular degeneration (AMD).**

Neovascular glaucoma: A type of glaucoma that sometimes occurs in people with retinal vascular disease, particularly diabetic retinopathy.

Night myopia: A condition in which visual acuity drops sharply in dim light.

Nonarteritic ischemic optic neuropathy: A condition, resulting from a painless swelling of the optic nerve, that is the most common cause of sudden vision loss in people 60 and older.

Nonproliferative (background) retinopathy: The mild form of diabetic retinopathy, characterized by a narrowing or weakening of small blood vessels in the eye.

Normal-tension glaucoma: A condition in which people with glaucomatous damage to the optic nerve have normal intraocular pressure.

Nuclear sclerosis: Descriptive of a type of cataract in which the nucleus gradually becomes more dense and opaque.

Ocular surface disease (OSD): A condition, characterized by excess tearing and eye irritation, that sometimes occurs in people with arthritis.

Opacity: The clouded area that forms in the normally transparent lens of the eye, eventually forming a cataract.

Open-angle glaucoma: The most common type of glaucoma in which fluid drains too slowly out of the eye.

Ophthalmologist: A physician (M.D. or D.O.) with special training and skill to diagnose and treat all diseases of the eye.

Ophthalmoscope: An instrument used in eye examinations to give a clear view of the retina, including the macula.

Optician: An eye care specialist trained to grind and formulate corrective lenses prescribed by an ophthalmologist or optometrist.

Optic nerve: The bundle of nerves at the back of the eye that carries images from the retina to the brain.

Optic neuritis: Inflammation of the optic nerve.

Optometrist: A doctor of optometry (O.D.) trained to refract the eye, diagnose disorders and sometimes treat them with drugs, but not to perform surgery.

Orbit: The bony socket in which the eye rests and that mostly encloses it.

Orthokeratology: A practice in which rigid contact lenses are applied in a series of sizes, to alter the shape of the cornea.

Orthoptics: A form of vision therapy often used to treat strabismus and amblyopia.

Perimetry: A measurement of peripheral vision that is an early-detector test for glaucoma.

Peripheral vision: The vision at the sides of a person's visual field; better known as side vision.

Phacoemulsification (PE): A variation of the extracapsular cataract extraction procedure in which the nucleus of the cataract is fragmented by ultrasound and aspirated from the eye.

Phorometer: An instrument, used in combination with a retinoscope, that contains a wide variety of optical lenses to help determine the appropriate prescription.

Photocoagulation: A laser treatment in which destructive blood vessels are sealed off and destroyed.

Photokeratitis: A painful and possibly vision-threatening condition in which the cornea is burned from intense light sources.

Photoreceptors: Those cells in the retina that convert light into electrical impulses that reach the optic nerve.

Photorefractive keratectomy (PRK): A procedure in which a laser is used to reshape the cornea, usually to correct for myopia.

Pinguecula: A yellowish bump on the eye, caused by a deposit of protein and fat.

Pneumatic retinopexy: A surgical procedure, to repair a retinal detachment, in which a gas bubble is injected into the vitreous space inside the eye.

Posterior capsular opacification: A common consequence of cataract surgery, in which the eye's posterior capsule clouds over, blurring vision.

Posterior subcapsular (PSC) cataract: A type of cataract, more common in people with diabetes, in which the opacity is centered on the back, or posterior, surface of the lens.

Potential vision testing: Tests used to determine whether the significant cause of visual impairment is a cataract or another eye problem.

Presbyopia: The gradual loss of flexibility of the lens inside the eye as a person ages, making it increasingly difficult to focus at close range.

Proliferative retinopathy: The most severe form of diabetic retinopathy, in which new blood vessels proliferate in the eye.

Proliferative vitreoretinopathy (PVR): A condition that sometimes occurs in people with diabetic retinopathy, characterized by the development of membranes on the retina, with reopening of retinal breaks, recurrent detachment and high risk for blindness.

Pseudoexotropia: The appearance of exotropia in very young children, due to widely set eyes and excess skin around the bridge of the nose.

Pseudostrabismus: The appearance of strabismus in very young children, due to a broad bridge of the nose and extra eyelid skin.

Pterygium: A fleshy growth resulting from the conjunctiva growing into the cornea.

Ptosis: A condition in which the upper eyelid droops over the eye.

Puncta: The small holes in the upper and lower lids, near the nose, through which tears drain.

Pupil: The "black" opening at the center of the iris.

Radial keratotomy (RK): A surgical procedure, to correct nearsightedness, in which incisions are made in the cornea to flatten it.

Refraction: The normal bending of light waves by the eyes to focus; also, the test carried out by eye care specialists to measure visual acuity.

Refractive errors: Common eye disorders in which the shape of the eye does not permit it to refract, or bend, light rays properly and thus produces a blurred image.

Retina: The nerve layer at the back of the eye that senses light and helps send images to the brain.

Retinal pigment epithelium (RPE): The extreme outer layer of the retina.

Retinitis pigmentosa (RP): A degenerative retinal condition that is inherited and causes slow but progressive loss of vision.

Retinoblastoma: A rare, malignant tumor originating in the retina, usually in very young children.

Retinopathy: Disease of blood vessels in the retina.

Retinopathy of prematurity (ROP): A condition developed by some premature infants in which abnormal blood vessels and scar tissue grow over the retina.

Retinoscope: Optical instrument used in examination to detect refractive errors in the eye; this is done by shining a light into the eye and noting how it is reflected as different lenses are placed in front of the eye.

Retinotomy: An operation to reattach the macula, in which the surgeon makes a "relaxing" incision of the peripheral retina.

Retrolental fibroplasia: See **Retinopathy of prematurity (ROP)**.

Rods: Cells in the retina that are responsible for peripheral vision.

Sclera: The tough, white, fibrous protective outer layer of the eye.

Scleral buckling: Surgery to repair a detached retina, in which a silicone band is wrapped around the eye.

Sclerostomy: See **Trabeculectomy**.

Secondary glaucoma: A type of glaucoma that can occur as the result of an eye injury, inflammation or tumor.

Sjögren's syndrome: A type of dry eye associated with arthritis and a drying of mucous membranes.

Slit lamp: Optical instrument, used in examination, that focuses a vertical beam on the eye, giving a view of a thin section of tissue.

Snellen chart: The traditional eye chart used to measure visual acuity; named for its ophthalmologist inventor.

Specular photographic microscopy: Testing that evaluates the ability of the cornea to withstand cataract surgery.

Stereopsis: The ability to see objects in three dimensions; also, depth perception. Also called stereoscopic vision.

Stereoscopic vision: See **Stereopsis**.

Strabismus: A disorder in which the eyes are misaligned and point in different directions; commonly called crossed eyes.

Sty: An pimplelike infection of one of the small glands on the edge of the eyelid.

Subconjunctival hemorrhage: A broken blood vessel just under the conjunctiva; it produces a bright red spot on the eye.

Tonometry: A measurement of intraocular pressure that is the primary test for glaucoma.

Torn retina: A condition in which a tear or hole in the retina allows fluid from the vitreous cavity to leak in.

Trabecular meshwork: The system of tiny drainage canals, all around the outer edge of the iris, through which fluid drains from the eye.

Trabeculectomy: A microsurgical procedure, to control glaucoma, in which a tiny opening is made in the sclera to facilitate drainage of fluid from the eye.

Trabeculoplasty: A procedure to control glaucoma in which a laser is used to open blocked drainage canals.

Trachoma: A serious corneal infection typically caused by chlamydia, a sexually transmitted disease.

Type-I diabetes: Type of diabetes in which the body loses the capacity to produce insulin. Also called insulin-dependent diabetes or juvenile-onset diabetes.

Type-II diabetes: Type of diabetes in which the body produces some insulin, but that insulin is for some reason ineffective. It usually appears after age 40 and is associated with obesity. Also called non-insulin-dependent diabetes or adult-onset diabetes.

Usher syndrome: An inherited disorder in which retinitis pigmentosa is combined with severe hearing loss.

VF-14: A visual function index that measures cataract-related impairment based on a person's ability to perform 14 everyday activities.

Vision therapy: Exercises and training routines based on the notion that vision is learned and that the brain can be trained to give the correct instructions to the muscles of the eye.

Visual acuity: How well one sees at given distances, typically measured by the Snellen chart.

Visual field: The entire view, both central and peripheral, that's visible when the eye is looking in any given direction.

Vitrectomy: A surgical procedure in which vitreous body and blood are removed and are replaced with gas or other substances.

Vitreous humor: The clear jellylike fluid that fills the inside of the eye.

Wet AMD: See **Neovascular AMD**. See also **Age-related macular degeneration (AMD)**.

YAG (yttrium aluminum garnet) laser capsulotomy: A procedure to restore vision in cataract patients who develop posterior capsular opacification.

Zonules: The numerous thin strands that connect the ciliary muscles to the lens of the eye.

SUGGESTED READING

Agency for Health Care Policy and Research. "Cataract in Adults: Management of Functional Impairment (Clinical Practice Guideline)." Publication No. AHCPR 93-0542. Rockville, Md.: Agency for Health Care Policy and Research, Public Health Service, U.S. Department of Health and Human Services, February 1993.

D'Amico, Donald J., M.D. "Disease of the Retina." *New England Journal of Medicine* 331 (July 14, 1994): 95-106.

Javitt, Jonathan C., M.D., M.P.H., et al. "Undertreatment of Glaucoma Among Black Americans." *New England Journal of Medicine* 325 (November 14, 1991): 1418-22.

Levin, Leonard A., M.D., Ph.D. "Ophthalmology." *Journal of the American Medical Association* 273 (June 7, 1995): 1703-5.

Mares-Perlman, Julie A., Ph.D., et al. "Diet and Nuclear Lens Opacities." *American Journal of Epidemiology* 141 (1995): 322-34.

Mares-Perlman, Julie A., Ph.D., et al. "Dietary Fat and Age-Related Maculopathy." *Archives of Ophthalmology* 113 (June 1995): 743-8.

Quigley, Harry A., M.D. "Open-Angle Glaucoma." *New England Journal of Medicine* 328 (April 15, 1993): 1097-1106.

Seddon, Johanna M., M.D., et al. "Dietary Carotenoids, Vitamins A, C, and E, and Advanced Age-Related Macular Degeneration." *Journal of the American Medical Association* 272 (November 9, 1994): 1413-20.

Shulman, Julius. *Cataracts*. New York: St. Martin's Press, 1995.

Steinberg, Earl P., M.D., M.P.P., et al. "The VF-14: An Index of Functional Impairment in Patients With Cataract." *Archives of Ophthalmology* 112 (May 1994): 630-8.

Tichelli, Andre, M.D., et al. "Cataract Formation After Bone Marrow Transplantation." *Annals of Internal Medicine* 119 (December 15, 1993): 1175-9.

Vajdos, Margaret A., M.D., et al. "Does Normalization of Blood Glucose Reduce the Complications of Diabetes?" *Southern Medical Journal* 88 (March 1995): 372-6.

Appendix:
TYPES OF EYE DEVICES

GLASSES

Ophthalmic lenses, or glasses, are commonly used to correct
vision. They are also sometimes used as protective devices in
sports or industrial settings.

Types of Lens Materials

Glass. Glass is the oldest and best material available for optics.
  It is scratch-resistant, and can be treated to increase its
  impact resistance. Its major drawback is weight—about
  twice that of a plastic lens.

Plastic (hard resin). Plastic lenses are lighter than glass
  lenses. They are less likely to break than glass, but scratch
  more easily unless treated. Plastic lenses can be tinted to
  almost any color or shade.

High index. These lenses—a result of modern technology—
  bend light differently so that stronger corrections are thinner
  than when made in conventional materials. They are available in glass or plastic, although glass tends to be heavier
  and thicker. They absorb potentially harmful ultraviolet light
  and can be tinted to any color or shade.

Polycarbonate. This impact-resistant material—first used for
  bulletproof windows in the 1960s—is used most often for
  active people and young people. The lenses are light, absorb
  potentially harmful ultraviolet light and can be tinted.

Photosensitive. These lenses, made of glass or plastic, darken in the sun (the effect of near ultraviolet rays on crystals within the lenses). The photosensitive effect is permanent, and will not fade or wear out. They are available in a variety of indoor and outdoor tints.

Types of Lens Designs

Single-vision lenses. These lenses correct vision at one distance only. They can be made of any lens material.

Bifocals. Bifocals act as a dual optical system. They correct vision at two distances, for example distance and near (reading) vision.

Straight top bifocals. Also called flat top bifocals, these have a bifocal portion (usually 25 millimeters across) marked by a visible horizontal line. The optical center is close to the segment line, so there is a minimal amount of distortion, or "image jump," when the wearer switches from distance to near vision.

Round bifocals. These have a round segment that is less visible than the straight top. However, there is more "image jump" when the wearer switches from distance to near vision.

Franklin style bifocals. Also called straight-across or executive bifocals, these have a large ridge running across the entire lens. It provides a wide field of vision and close to no "image jump" for the wearer. The lens is heavier and thicker than other types of bifocal lens design.

Trifocals. Trifocals correct at three distances, for example, distance vision, reading vision and an intermediate distance (arm's length). They are usually available in the same designs as bifocals are.

Progressive (no-line) bifocals. These lenses progressively correct vision from distance to near, offering continuous vision without segment lines. However, they must be fitted carefully, and there may be distortions. They look like single-vision lenses, and are available in any material.

Aspheric. These lightweight lenses are used for stronger corrections. They are thinner than conventional lenses, which may appear to bulge and often distort the wearer's face. Aspheric lenses minimize distortion and provide better clarity at the edges of the lenses. They can used as single-vision or bifocal lenses.

Occupational. Special lenses can be created for workers whose occupations (dentistry, jewelry work, accounting, et cetera) impose demanding visual requirements. Common occupational lenses include the double-segment bifocal, which has a second bifocal segment at the top of the lens, and the quadrifocal, which has a trifocal as its bottom segment and a bifocal as its top segment.

Polarized. These lenses eliminate reflective glare. They are often the choice of drivers, fishers and hunters, and are also available as a feature of sunglasses.

Sunglasses. Sunglasses—lenses tinted green, gray or brown—should screen out at least 99 percent of potentially harmful ultraviolet rays, and 75 to 90 percent of visible light. Sunglasses may be polarized to reduce glare, or may be photo-sensitive, meaning they darken according to the amount of light available. Mirrored sunglasses reflect light and are best used against glare from snow or water.

Other Options

Antireflective. This coating helps reduce eye fatigue and may be appropriate for computer operators or those who drive at night.

Scratch protection. A special coating can be applied to plastic lenses to help prevent scratches.

Ultraviolet protection. Because ultraviolet rays from the sun are potentially harmful to the eyes, plastic lenses may be treated to block ultraviolet light. High index and poly-carbonate lenses may have built-in ultraviolet protection.

CONTACT LENSES

Contact lenses are thin sheets of plastic that are made to fit the cornea, the front surface of the eye. The lenses correct vision as glasses do, while providing good peripheral vision and reducing distortion. Because they do not fog up or fall off, contacts are well-suited for those with an active lifestyle as well as those who do not wish to wear glasses for cosmetic reasons. The amount of daily care and cleaning varies with the type of lens.

Hard lenses. Hard lenses are made of inflexible plastics that oxygen cannot penetrate; instead, oxygen passes around and underneath the lenses. They provide sharp vision and correct most vision problems. Although the most durable of all types of contact lenses, these lenses require daily cleaning, rinsing and disinfecting. They often require a longer adaptation period and consistent wear to maintain adaptation and comfort.

Rigid gas-permeable (RGP) lenses. RGP lenses are made of slightly flexible plastic that allows oxygen to pass through to the eyes. They are durable, provide excellent vision and are comfortable to wear after a short adaptation period. Most wearers are able to switch between RGP lenses and glasses without blurred vision. But constant wear is necessary to maintain the comfort of the lenses, and they can slip off the center of the eye easily. They must cleaned, rinsed and disinfected daily.

Soft lenses. Soft lenses are created from many different plastics that allow oxygen to pass through the lens to nourish the eye. These lenses offer easy adaptation and comfortable wear usually from the start. They offer the wearer the ability to switch from contacts to glasses without blurred vision and infrequent wear without readaptation. Their close fit makes them less likely to be dislodged and less likely to have anything trapped underneath. However, soft lenses don't correct all vision problems and may not provide the sharp vision that some other lenses do. They need to be replaced periodically as recommended by your eye care practitioner. Daily-wear soft lenses must be cleaned, rinsed and disinfected daily.

Daily-wear disposable lenses. These are soft lenses that are thrown away at the end of each day, eliminating cleaning and care.

Extended-wear lenses. These are RGP or soft plastic lenses that can be worn up to seven days without being removed. These do not correct all vision problems. They require two to four office visits a year for follow-up care and may need to be replaced about once a year. They must be cleaned, rinsed and disinfected every seven days.

Extended-wear disposable lenses. Extended-wear disposable lenses are soft lenses that are worn for one to seven days, then thrown away. They require little care and reduce the risk of eye infection, since they are frequently disposed. They do not correct all vision problems.

Planned replacement lenses. These are soft lenses that are replaced according to a schedule, most often every two weeks, monthly or quarterly. They require less cleaning than other lenses and reduce the risk of eye infection. They do not correct all vision problems and may not provide vision as sharp as RGP lenses.

Special designs. Lenses can be specially adapted to correct for high amounts of astigmatism, or be adapted for use as bifocal lenses. These specially designed lenses are available in RGP and soft lens materials.

Tinted lenses. Most contact lenses are available as colored lenses. While some are lightly tinted to help in locating lost lenses, others are tinted to enhance or change eye color.

Source: American Optometric Association.

INDEX

A

A-scan
  cataract surgery and, 116
  defined, 116, 159
Accidents, eye injuries and, 145
Accommodative esotropia,
  defined, 41-42, 159
Acetazolamide (Diamox),
  glaucoma and, 137
Acquired immune deficiency
  syndrome (AIDS). *See* AIDS
Age
  cataracts and, 103-104, 107
  dry eye and, 60
  eye exam frequency and, 21
  glaucoma and, 131-132
  macular degeneration and,
    68-69
  myopia and, 26
  night myopia and, 64-65
  strabismus and, 36
Age-related macular degeneration.
  See AMD
Aging eyes. *See* Presbyopia
AIDS
  CMV (cytomegalovirus) retinitis
    and, 96-98

detached retina and, 85
eye exam and, 98
Alcohol, cataracts and, 109
Aldose reductase
  defined, 82, 159
  diabetic retinopathy and, 82
Amblyopia
  causes, 43
  defined, 43, 159
  diagnosis, 43-44
  ptosis and, 56
  treatment, 43-44
AMD. *See also* Dry AMD;
    Neovascular AMD
  defined, 69, 159
  diagnosis, 72
  genetics and, 70
  incidence, 69
  prevention, 73-74
  risk factors, 69-70, 73-74
  symptoms, 71, 91
Amsler grid
  AMD and, 72
  defined, 72, 159
Anemia, conjunctivitis and, 53-54
Antibiotics
  cataract surgery, 122

179

conjunctivitis, 50
corneal infections, 54
Antidepressants, dry eye and, 61
Antihistamines, dry eye and, 61
Antioxidants, glaucoma and, 143
Aphakia, defined, 119, 159
Aqueous humor, defined, 12, 159
ARMD. *See* AMD
Arteriosclerosis, optic nerve and, 147
Arthritis
    dry eye and, 61
    ocular surface disease (OSD) and, 59
    rheumatoid, effects, 54
Artificial tears, dry eye and, 62
Aspirin
    cataracts and, 110
    diabetic retinopathy and, 81
Astigmatism
    amblyopia and, 43
    defined, 25, 29, 159
    photorefractive keratotomy (PRK), 32
    ptosis and, 56
    radial keratotomy (RK), 31, 119
Atherosclerosis, conjunctivitis and, 53-54

B

Background retinopathy. *See* Nonproliferative retinopathy
Bacterial infection, cataract surgery and, 122
Beta blockers
    dry eye and, 61
    glaucoma and, 137, 138
Betaxolol (Betoptic), glaucoma and, 137
Betoptic. *See* Betaxolol (Betoptic)

Bifocals. *See also* Glasses
    refractive errors and, 29
Binocular vision
    defined, 15
    depth perception and, 15
Biomicroscope. *See* Slit lamp
Bleb, defined, 140-141, 160
Blepharitis, defined, 50-51, 160
Blindness
    AMD and, 69
    diabetic retinopathy and, 79, 80
    glaucoma and, 127, 131
    legal. *See* Legal blindness
    low vision vs., 16
    macular degeneration and, 67, 68
    retinal donor program and, 68
    retinitis pigmentosa (RP) and, 90-91
    scleral buckling and, 89
    sleep-wake cycles and, 16-17
    Usher syndrome and, 93
Blocked tear duct. *See* Dacryostenosis
Blood pressure
    conjunctivitis and, 53-54
    glaucoma and, 132, 143
Bone marrow transplantation, cataracts and, 108
Botox. *See* Botulinum toxin-A
Botulinum toxin-A, strabismus and, 41
Brain tumors, strabismus and, 35, 36

C

Capsule, defined, 12, 160
Carbonic anhydrase inhibitors
    defined, 137, 160
    glaucoma and, 137, 138

Carotenoids, defined, 74, 160
Cataracts
  aphakia and, 119-120
  causes, 103-104, 107-110
  defined, 103, 160
  diabetes and, 83-84
  diagnosis, 106
  generally, 16
  glaucoma and, 132
  incidence, 103
  lasers, generally, 117
  pneumatic retinopexy and, 89
  prevention, 109-110
  progression, 106
  ptosis and, 56
  scleral buckling and, 89
  strabismus and, 35
  surgery
    complications, 122-123
    delay between operations, 125
    effects, 121
    government guidelines, 112-113
    HCFA and, 111-112
    incidence, 110-111
    lenses, 119-120
    preoperative tests, 113-117
    reasons for, 116
    recovery, 121
    safety, 122
    types, 117
  types, 104
  vision effects, 105
Central island of vision, effects, 19
Central vision, cone cells and, 14
Cerebral palsy, strabismus and, 35
Children, eye exam recommendations, 21
Chlamydia, effects, 53

Choroid, defined, 12, 160
Choroid tumors, choroidal melanoma, 99
Choroidal melanoma
  defined, 99, 160
  incidence, 99
  symptoms/treatment, 99
Ciliary muscles, defined, 13, 160
Closed-angle glaucoma. *See* Glaucoma, closed-angle
Closed-circuit TV (CCTV), low vision and, 151
CMV (cytomegalovirus) retinitis
  AIDS and, 96-98
  defined, 67, 96, 160
  treatment, 96-98
Color blindness
  defined, 62-63
  risk factors, 63
  treatment, 63
Color vision, cone cells and, 14-15
Cones, defined, 14, 159
Congenital glaucoma. *See* Glaucoma, congenital
Conjunctiva, defined, 11, 161
Conjunctival tumors, treatment, 147
Conjunctivitis
  causes, 48
  defined, 47-48, 161
  symptoms, 48-49
  treatment, 49
Contact lenses
  eye exam recommendations, 21
  keratoconus and, 148
  opticians and, 22
  refractive errors and, 29
  slit-lamp exam and, 20
  types, 176-177

Contrast-sensitivity testing, cataract surgery and, 113

Contrast sensitivity, defined, 65, 161

Convergence insufficiency, defined, 42, 161

Cornea, defined, 11, 12, 161

Corneal degenerative disease, eye donors and, 149

Corneal disease, diabetes and, 83-84

Corneal dystrophy, defined, 148

Corneal infections. *See also* Herpes simplex virus; Herpetic keratitis; Trachoma
generally, 51-52
treatment, 54

Corneal transplant
corneal infections and, 54
pros/cons, 149-150

Cortex, defined, 12, 161

Cortical cataract, defined, 103, 161

Corticosteroids
glaucoma and, 132
optic neuritis, 55

Costs, cost-free eye care, 152

Crossed eyes. *See* Strabismus

Cryotherapy
defined, 86, 161
detached retina, 89
retinoblastoma, 100
retinopathy of prematurity (ROP), 101-102
torn retina, 86-87

Cystoid macular edema, cataract surgery and, 122

Cytomegalovirus retinitis. *See* CMV (cytomegalovirus) retinitis

Cytovene. *See* Ganciclovir (Cytovene)

D

Dacryocystorhinostomy, defined, 59

Dacryostenosis
defined, 58, 161
treatment, 59

Depth perception, stereopsis and, 15

Detached retina
complications, 89-90
defined, 67, 84, 161
diagnosis, 86
incidence, 85
risk factors, 85
symptoms, 86
treatment, 87-90

Diabetes
cataracts and, 83-84, 104, 107
conjunctivitis and, 53-54
corneal disease and, 83-84
corneal infections and, 53-54
detached retina and, 85
eye exam recommendations, 81
glaucoma and, 130, 132
pregnancy and, 82-83
ptosis and, 56
retinopathy. *See* Diabetic retinopathy
strabismus and, 36
types, 77, 169

Diabetic retinopathy
defined, 67, 76, 161
diabetes, generally, 76-78
early symptoms, 81
eye exam recommendations, 81
incidence, 76
neovascular glaucoma and, 130
nonproliferative, 78
prevention, 81-82

proliferative, 78
treatment, 79-80
Diamox. *See* Acetazolamide (Diamox)
Diet
AMD and, 73-74
cataracts and, 107, 109-110
glaucoma and, 143
Dipivefrin (Propine), glaucoma and, 137
Diplopia
defined, 35, 161
strabismus and, 38
Distorted vision. *See* Astigmatism
Diuretics, dry eye and, 61
Donors, eye, 68, 149-150
Dorzolamide hydrochloride (Trusopt), glaucoma and, 137
Double vision. *See* Diplopia
Down syndrome
keratoconus and, 148
strabismus and, 35
Drusen, defined, 70, 161
Dry AMD
defined, 70, 161
treatment, 72
Dry eye
causes, 60-61
defined, 58, 60-61, 162
diagnosis, 61

E

Eclipse, solar, photokeratitis and, 148
Ectropion, defined, 57, 162
Electroretinogram (ERG), defined, 92-93
Endophthalmitis, defined, 122
Endothelium, defined, 114, 162
Entropion, defined, 57, 162

Epifrin. *See* Epinephrine (Epifrin)
Epinephrine (Epifrin), glaucoma and, 137, 138
Esotropia
accommodative, defined, 41-42, 159
defined, 35, 162
surgery, 38-40
Estrogen, dry eye and, 60, 62
Exercise, glaucoma and, 143
Exotropia. *See also* Pseudoexotropia
defined, 35, 162
surgery, 38, 40
Extracapsular surgery
defined, 118
phacoemulsification vs., 118-119
Eye, composition, 11-12
Eye care, cost-free, 152
Eye doctors. *See* Ophthalmologist; Optician; Optometrist
Eye donors, 68, 149-150
Eye injuries, prevention, 145
Eye treatment centers, ophthalmology hospitals, 155-157
Eye tumors, ptosis and, 56
Eyedrops
eye exam and, 20
myopia prevention, 33-34
open-angle glaucoma and, 136
Eyelid, role, 16
Eyelid tumors, treatment, 147

F

Farsightedness. *See* Hyperopia; Presbyopia
Field expanders, low vision and, 151
5-Fluorouracil, microsurgery and, 141

Flashes, light, causes, 47
Floaters
    causes, 46
    complications, 46-47
    defined, 45, 162
Fluorescein
    defined, 60, 162
    dry eye and, 61
    excessive tearing and, 60
Fluorescein angiogram, AMD and, 72
Foscarnet (Foscavir), CMV (cyto-megalovirus) retinitis and, 96-97
Foscavir. See Foscarnet (Foscavir)
Fovea, defined, 14, 162
Fuchs' dystrophy, defined, 148, 162

G

Galactosemia, defined, 104, 162
Ganciclovir (Cytovene), CMV (cytomegalovirus) retinitis and, 96-98
Gene therapy, retinitis pigmentosa (RP) and, 95
Genetics
    AMD and, 70
    glaucoma and, 132
    macular degeneration and, 70
    retinitis pigmentosa (RP) and, 90-91
    Usher syndrome and, 93
Glare testing, cataract surgery and, 113
Glasses
    lens designs, types, 174-175
    lens materials, types, 173-174
    plus, accommodative esotropia and, 42
Glaucoma
    causes, 130-132
    closed-angle
        defined, 128, 160
        treatment, 141-143
    congenital
        defined, 130, 160
        treatment, 141-143
    defined, 127, 162
    detached retina and, 85
    diagnosis, 133-135
    exam recommendations, 134-135
    eye exam frequency and, 21
    generally, 16
    incidence, 131
    intraocular pressure (IOP) and, 124, 127-130, 132-133, 135-136, 143
    neovascular, defined, 130, 164
    normal-tension, defined, 130, 164
    open-angle
        causes, 129
        defined, 128, 165
        treatment, 136
    optic nerve and, 20
    peripheral vision and, 19
    prevention/control, 143
    scleral buckling and, 89
    secondary, defined, 130, 168
    treatment
        laser therapy, 139-140
        medications, 137-139
        microsurgery, 140-142
        reasons for, 135-136
    types, 127, 130
    YAG laser capsulotomy and, 124
Gonioscopy, defined, 134, 162
Gonorrhea, conjunctivitis and, 48
Growth factors, retinitis pigmentosa (RP) and, 95

H

Handheld magnifiers, low vision and, 150

HCFA, cataract surgery and, 111-112

Health Care Financing Administration (HCFA). *See* HCFA

Health maintenance organizations (HMOs). *See* HMOs

Hemorrhage, subconjunctival, defined, 50, 169

Herpes simplex virus, effects, 52-53

Herpetic keratitis, defined, 52, 163

HIV, eye exam and, 98

HMOs, optometrists vs. ophthalmologists, 24

Hormone replacement therapy, dry eye and, 62

Human immunodeficiency virus (HIV). *See* HIV

Hydrocephalus, strabismus and, 35

Hydrogen peroxide, cataracts and, 110

Hyperopia
amblyopia and, 43
defined, 25, 28-29, 163

I

Informational and mutual-aid groups, 153-154

Intracapsular surgery, defined, 117

Intraocular lens (IOL), defined, 116, 163

Intraocular pressure (IOP)
defined, 124, 163
glaucoma and, 124, 127-130, 132-133, 135-136, 143

normal levels, 133

IOL. *See* Intraocular lens (IOL)

IOP. *See* Intraocular pressure (IOP)

Iridectomy, defined, 140, 163

Iridotomy, defined, 141-142, 163

Iris, defined, 12, 163

K

Keratoconus, defined, 148, 163

Keratometer
cataract surgery and, 116
defined, 116, 163

Keratotomy. *See also* Mini-RK; Photorefractive keratotomy (PRK); Radial keratotomy (RK)
cataract surgery and, 119

L

Lacrimal gland, defined, 15, 163

Lacrimal sac, defined, 15, 163

Lasers. *See also* Surgery; Trabeculoplasty
AMD and, 72-73
detached retina and, 89
open-angle glaucoma and, 136, 139-140
retinopathy of prematurity (ROP), 101-102
torn retina and, 86-87
YAG laser capsulotomy, 123

Latanoprost, glaucoma and, 137

Lazy eye. *See* Amblyopia

Legal blindness
defined, 18, 163
peripheral vision and, 19

Lens
defined, 12, 163
parts, 104

Levator
    defined, 56, 163
    ptosis and, 56
Low vision
    blindness vs., 16
    defined, 16, 164
    optical aids, 150-151
Lyme disease, effects, 54

M

Macula, defined, 12, 164
Macular degeneration. *See also*
    AMD
    defined, 67, 68, 164
    genetics and, 70
Macular edema
    defined, 78, 164
    treatment, 79
Magnifying spectacles, low vision
    and, 150
Marijuana, glaucoma and, 143
Menopause, dry eye and, 60, 62
Methazolamide (Neptazane),
    glaucoma and, 137
Microaneurysms, defined, 78, 164
Migraine, ocular, 47
Milk intolerance, cataracts and,
    104
Mini-RK
    defined, 31-32
    pros/cons, 31-32
Miotics, glaucoma and, 137, 138,
    164
Multiple sclerosis, effects, 54, 55
Musicians, glaucoma and, 132
Myasthenia gravis, strabismus
    and, 36
Myopia. *See also* Night myopia
    age and, 26
    amblyopia and, 43

cataract surgery and, 117
corneal ring surgery, 33
defined, 23, 25, 26, 164
detached retina and, 85
glaucoma and, 132
mini-RK, 32
photorefractive keratotomy
    (PRK), 32
prevention
    eyedrops, medicated, 33-34
    neuropeptides, growth-
        stimulating, 34
    vision therapy, 34-35
radial keratotomy (RK), 30-32
risk factors, 27-28

N

Nearsightedness. *See* Myopia
Neovascular AMD, defined, 71,
    164
Neovascular glaucoma. *See*
    Glaucoma, neovascular
Neptazane. *See* Methazolamide
    (Neptazane)
Neurological disorders,
    strabismus and, 35, 36
Neuropeptides, growth-
    stimulating, myopia prevention
    with, 34
Night blindness, generally, 65
Night myopia
    causes, 64
    defined, 64, 164
Night vision. *See also* Night
    myopia
    defined, 64
    night vision aids (NVAs), 151
Nonarteritic ischemic optic
    neuropathy
    defined, 146, 164
    treatment, 146

Nonproliferative retinopathy, defined, 78, 164

Normal-tension glaucoma. *See* Glaucoma, normal-tension

Normal vision, defined, 18

Nuclear sclerosis, defined, 104, 164

O

Obesity, conjunctivitis and, 53-54

Occupational hazards
cataracts, 108
glaucoma, 108

Ocular surface disease (OSD), defined, 59, 165

Ocusert. *See* Pilocarpine (Ocusert)

Ocuvite, AMD and, 74

Opacity, defined, 103, 165

Open-angle glaucoma. *See* Glaucoma, open-angle

Ophthalmologist
defined, 165
education requirements, 21-22
Snellen, Herman, 17
vs. optometrist, 22-24

Ophthalmology, treatment centers, 155-157

Ophthalmoscope, defined, 20, 165

Ophthalmoscopy, defined, 133

Optic nerve
arteriosclerosis and, 147
defined, 11, 12, 165

Optic nerve compression, nonarteritic ischemic optic neuropathy and, 146

Optic neuritis
defined, 54, 165
symptoms/treatment, 55

Optician, defined, 22, 165

Optometrist
defined, 22, 165
education requirements, 22

Orbit, defined, 11, 165

Orbital tumors, treatment, 147

Orthokeratology, defined, 30, 165

Orthoptics, defined, 41, 165

P

Pain relievers, dry eye and, 61

Patch, eye
amblyopia, 44
corneal infections, 54

PE. *See* Phacoemulsification (PE)

Perimetry, defined, 134, 165

Peripheral vision
defined, 14, 165
eye exam and, 18-19

Phacoemulsification, extracapsular surgery vs., 118-119

Phacoemulsification (PE), defined, 117

Phorometer, defined, 20, 166

Photocoagulation
AMD and, 72-73
defined, 72, 166
diabetic retinopathy and, 79, 80
macular edema and, 79
retinopathy of prematurity (ROP) and, 101-102

Photokeratitis, defined, 148, 166

Photoreceptor cells
defined, 13-14, 166
retinitis pigmentosa (RP) and, 90

Photorefractive keratotomy (PRK)
defined, 32-33, 166
pros/cons, 32-33

Pilocarpine hydrochloride (Pilopine HS), glaucoma and, 137

Pilocarpine (Ocusert), glaucoma and, 137

Pilopine HS. See Pilocarpine hydrochloride (Pilopine HS)

Pinguecula
defined, 65, 166
treatment, 66

Plus glasses, accommodative esotropia and, 42

Pneumatic retinopexy
defined, 87, 166
detached retina and, 87-89

Posterior capsular opacification
defined, 123, 166
treatment, 123

Posterior subcapsular (PSC) cataract
defined, 104, 166
symptoms, 105

Potential vision testing
cataract surgery and, 113-114
defined, 113, 166

Pregnancy, diabetic retinopathy and, 82-83

Premature babies, complications, 100-101

Presbyopia
cataract surgery and, 117
defined, 25, 28-29, 166
glaucoma and, 132

Prisms
amblyopia and, 44
strabismus and, 41

Proliferative retinopathy, defined, 78-79, 166

Proliferative vitreoretinopathy (PVR)
defined, 89, 167
scleral buckling and, 89

Prostaglandin, glaucoma and, 137, 139

Proteins, AMD and, 75-76

PSC cataract. See Posterior subcapsular (PSC) cataract

Pseudoexotropia, defined, 37, 167

Pseudostrabismus, defined, 37, 167

Pterygium
defined, 66, 167
treatment, 66

Ptosis
complications, 56
defined, 55-56, 167

Puncta, defined, 62, 167

Pupil, defined, 12, 167

PVR. See Proliferative vitreoretinopathy (PVR)

R

Race
diabetic retinopathy and, 82
glaucoma and, 131-132

Radial keratotomy (RK)
defined, 30-31, 167
pros/cons, 31-32

Radiation
cataracts and, 108
choroidal melanoma and, 99
retinoblastoma and, 100
tumors and, 147

Refraction, defined, 13, 167

Refractive errors. See also Astigmatism; Hyperopia; Myopia; Presbyopia
defined, 25, 167
incidence, 25-26

Research, eye donors and, 68

Retina
defined, 12, 167
detached. See Detached retina
generally, 67-68
torn. See Torn retina

Retina tumors, retinoblastoma, 98-100

Retinal cell transplantation, AMD and, 73

Retinal degenerative disease, eye donors and, 68

Retinal detachment. *See* Detached retina; Torn retina

Retinal pigment epithelium (RPE), defined, 12, 167

Retinitis pigmentosa (RP)
    defined, 65, 90, 167
    diagnosis, 92-93
    eye donors and, 68
    genetics, 90-91
    incidence, 90
    symptoms, 91-92
    treatment, 94-95
    Usher syndrome and, 93

Retinoblastoma
    defined, 99, 168
    incidence, 99, 168

Retinopathy of prematurity (ROP)
    causes, 101
    defined, 100, 168
    treatment, 101-102

Retinoscope, defined, 20, 168

Retinotomy, defined, 89, 168

Retrolental fibroplasia, defined, 100, 168

Rheumatoid arthritis, effects, 54

RK. *See* Radial keratotomy (RK)

Rods, defined, 14, 168

ROP. *See* Retinopathy of prematurity (ROP)

RP. *See* Retinitis pigmentosa (RP)

RPE. *See* Retinal pigment epithelium (RPE)

S

Sclera, defined, 11, 168

Scleral buckling
    defined, 87, 168
    detached retina and, 87-89

Sclerostomy, defined, 140, 160

Secondary glaucoma. *See* Glaucoma, secondary

Sickle-cell anemia
    defined, 102
    effects, 102

Sickle-cell retinopathy, effects, 102

Side vision. *See* Peripheral vision

Silicone oil, detached retina and, 88

Sjögren's syndrome, defined, 61, 168

Sleep-wake cycles, eye's role, 16-17

Sleeping pills, dry eye and, 61

Slit lamp, defined, 19-20, 160, 168

Slit-lamp exam
    cataracts, 106
    contact lenses, 20
    glaucoma, 134

Smoking
    cataracts and, 108
    glaucoma and, 143

Snellen, Herman, Snellen chart and, 17

Snellen chart
    cataracts and, 106
    defined, 17, 168

Specular photographic microscopy
    cataract surgery and, 113-114
    defined, 113, 168

Stereopsis, defined, 15, 169

Stereoscopic vision, defined, 43, 169

Steroids, cataracts and, 104, 108

Stitches, cataract surgery and, 118-119

Strabismus. *See also* Convergence insufficiency; Esotropia; Exotropia; Pseudoexotropia; Pseudostrabismus
age and, 36
defined, 35, 169
diagnosis, 37
diplopia and, 38
drug therapy, 41-42
incidence, 36
infants, 36-37
orthoptics, 41
prisms, 41
ptosis and, 56
risk factors, 35-36
surgery, 38-40
vision therapy, 23, 41-42

Stroke
ptosis and, 56
strabismus and, 36

Sty, defined, 51, 169

Subconjunctival hemorrhage, defined, 50, 169

Sunglasses, cataracts and, 109, 124

Sunlight, cataracts and, 108, 109, 124

Surgery. *See also* Lasers
adjustable-suture, 39
cataracts
complications, 122-123
delay between operations, 125
effects, 121
generally, 106-107
government guidelines, 112-113
HCFA and, 111-112
incidence, 110-111
lenses, 119-120
preoperative tests, 113-117
recovery, 121
safety, 122
types, 117
choroidal melanoma, 99
corneal ring, 33
corneal transplant, 149-150
microsurgery, glaucoma, 136, 140-141
mini-RK, 31-32
optic nerve compression, nonarteritic ischemic optic neuropathy and, 146
photorefractive keratotomy (PRK), 32-33
pneumatic retinopexy, detached retina, 87-89
radial keratotomy (RK), 30-32, 119
retinal cell transplantation, AMD, 73
retinoblastoma, 100
retinopathy of prematurity (ROP), 101-102
scleral buckling, detached retina, 87-89
tumors, 147
vitrectomy
detached retina, 87
diabetic retinopathy, 80
endophthalmitis, 122

Syphilis, effects, 54

T

Tear duct, blocked. *See* Dacryostenosis

Tearing, excessive. *See also* Dacryostenosis; Ocular surface disease (OSD)
causes, 58-59
diagnosis, 60

Tears
  artificial, dry eye and, 62
  role, 15
Telescopes, low vision and, 150
Thyroid disease, strabismus and, 36
Timolol (Timoptic), glaucoma and, 137
Timoptic. *See* Timolol (Timoptic)
Tonometry, defined, 133, 169
Torn retina
  cataract surgery and, 122
  defined, 67, 84, 169
  diagnosis, 86
  pneumatic retinopexy and, 89
  symptoms, 86
  treatment, 86-87
Trabecular meshwork, defined, 127, 169
Trabeculectomy
  defined, 140, 169
  effects, 141
Trabeculoplasty, defined, 139, 169
Trachoma, defined, 53, 169
Transplantation
  corneal, 54, 149-150
  retinal cell, AMD and, 73
Trauma
  cataracts and, 108
  eye injuries and, 145
  glaucoma and, 132
Treatment centers, ophthalmology hospitals, 155-157
Trifocals. *See also* Glasses
  refractive errors and, 29
Trusopt. *See* Dorzolamide hydrochloride (Trusopt)
Tumors
  brain, strabismus and, 35, 36
  choroid, choroidal melanoma, 99

conjunctival, treatment, 147
  eye, ptosis and, 56
  eyelid, treatment, 147
  orbital, treatment, 147
  retina, retinoblastoma, 98-100
Tunnel vision, effects, 19
20/20 vision, defined, 18
Two-eyed vision. *See* Binocular vision
Type-I diabetes, defined, 77, 169
Type-II diabetes, defined, 77, 169

U

Ultraviolet light, cataracts and, 108, 109, 124
Usher syndrome
  causes, 93
  defined, 67, 93, 169
  eye donors and, 68
  genetics and, 93
  retinitis pigmentosa (RP) and, 93
  treatment, 94-95

V

VF-14
  cataracts and, 114-115
  defined, 114, 170
Vision, mechanics, 13-15
Vision therapy
  amblyopia and, 44-45
  defined, 23, 170
  myopia prevention, 34-35
  ophthalmologists and, 24, 34, 41-42, 45
Visual acuity
  defined, 17, 170
  eye exam and, 17-18
Visual field, defined, 14, 170

Vitamins
  AMD and, 74
  vitamin A, cataracts and,
    109-110
  vitamin A palmitate
    retinitis pigmentosa (RP)
      and, 94-95
    Usher syndrome and, 94-95
  vitamin E, retinitis pigmentosa
    (RP) and, 95
Vitrectomy
  defined, 80, 170
  detached retina, 87
  diabetic retinopathy, 80
  endophthalmitis, 122
Vitreous humor, defined, 12, 170

W

Wet AMD
  defined, 70, 164, 170
  treatment, 72-73

X

X-rays, cataracts and, 108

Y

YAG laser capsulotomy
  complications, 123-124
  defined, 123, 170
  posterior capsular opacification
    and, 123
Yttrium aluminum garnet laser
  capsulotomy. *See* YAG laser
  capsulotomy

Z

Zinc, AMD and, 74-75
Zonules, defined, 108, 170